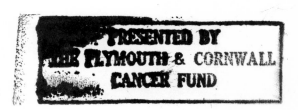
Nov 13th 1978

CROSS-SECTIONAL ANATOMY

Computed Tomography
and
Ultrasound Correlation

Barbara L. Carter, M.D.

Professor of Radiology, Tufts University School of Medicine; Chief, Computed Tomography of the Body; Chief, E.N.T. Radiology, New England Medical Center Hospital, Boston, Massachusetts

James Morehead, Ph.D.

Associate Professor of Anatomy; Associate Dean for Basic Science Affairs, Tufts University School of Medicine, Boston, Massachusetts

Samuel M. Wolpert, M.B.B.Ch., D.M.R.D.

Professor of Radiology, Tufts University School of Medicine; Chief of Neuroradiology and Cranial Computed Tomography, New England Medical Center Hospital, Boston, Massachusetts

Steven B. Hammerschlag, M.B.B.Ch., F.R.C.P. (C)

Instructor of Radiology, Tufts University School of Medicine; Assistant in Radiology, New England Medical Center Hospital, Boston, Massachusetts

Harry J. Griffiths, M.D.

Associate Professor, Tufts University School of Medicine; Senior Radiologist, New England Medical Center Hospital, Boston, Massachusetts

Paul C. Kahn, M.D.

Professor of Radiology, Tufts University School of Medicine; Chief of Nuclear Medicine and Ultrasound, New England Medical Center Hospital, Boston, Massachusetts

Body section diagrams adapted from A Cross-Section Anatomy, by Eycleshymer and Schoemaker

CROSS-SECTIONAL ANATOMY

Computed Tomography
and
Ultrasound Correlation

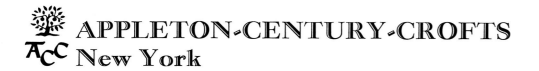 APPLETON-CENTURY-CROFTS
New York

Library of Congress Cataloging in Publication Data
Main entry under title:

Cross-sectional anatomy.

Includes index.
1. Anatomy, Human—Atlases. 2. Tomography—Atlases.
3. Diagnosis, Ultrasonic—Atlases. I. Carter, Barbara L.
QM25.C75   611′.0022′2   77–1299
ISBN 0–8385–1255–0

Prentice-Hall International, Inc., London
Prentice-Hall of Australia, Pty. Ltd., Sydney
Prentice-Hall of India Private Limited, New Delhi
Prentice-Hall of Japan, Inc., Tokyo
Prentice-Hall of Southeast Asia (Pte.) Ltd., Singapore
Whitehall Books Ltd., Wellington, New Zealand

PRINTED IN THE UNITED STATES OF AMERICA

Acknowledgments

The authors wish to express their deep appreciation and gratitude to the many people and organizations who helped in making this atlas possible. It was produced with the assistance of an educational grant from E. R. Squibb and Sons, Inc., and a grant from Ohio-Nuclear, Inc.

Much time and effort were expended by the members of the Department of Educational Media under the guidance of their chief, Mary B. Allen, who was our project coordinator. The medical photographers were Thomas Moon, assisted by Harry Maskell. Anthony Ross, assisted by Georgianna Powell, was responsible for the graphic art. And our special thanks to Karen Waldo, presently medical illustrator at the Medical College of Georgia, who did all the drawings of the head sections 1 through 7 and of the spine.

Many thanks are also due to the technicians involved with the CT scanning: Prudence Peart, R.T., Karen Payne, R.T., and David Green, R.T. X-rays of the actual specimens were taken by Theodore Grindle, R.T. Frederick Ingram, Chief Ultrasound Technologist, produced the echograms. We are deeply indebted to Donald Fisher, our own radiology engineer, and to Ken Hill of Ohio-Nuclear, Inc., for their help with the Delta Scanner.

Robert E. Paul, Jr., M.D., Chairman of the Department of Radiology and Jeffery P. Moore, M.D., Associate Chief, gave invaluable advice and moral support throughout the project. Innumerable other people including our secretaries under the supervision of Barbara Billings; Patricia Jayson, our own medical editor, assisted by Jeanne Leary; and Edward Cohen, our business manager, have helped in many and various ways in compiling the manuscript, organizing the material, and procuring the funds to make this Atlas a reality.

Last, but not least, our thanks are due to our publishers, Appleton-Century-Crofts (and particularly to Doreen Berne) for their patience, understanding, and ever-available advice.

Preface

This book draws heavily on the pioneering work, *A Cross-Section Anatomy,* by Eycleshymer and Schoemaker, first published by the D. Appleton Company in 1911. With the advent of ultrasonography and computerized tomography, there has been a renewed interest in atlases which display the human body in cross-section.

The first known reference to the use of cross-sectional anatomy was in the early part of the sixteenth century, when, according to Chamberlaine and Choulant, Leonardo da Vinci pictured median sagittal sections of the bodies of both the male and female; the sections were represented as extending from the level of the shoulder to the lower portion of the pelvis. The Flemish anatomist, André Vésale, was probably the first to depict transverse sections of the brain. In the seventeenth century, Vidius, Placentinus, Spieghel, Fludd, Bartholin, Vesling, de Graaf, and others depicted cross-sections of various parts of the body, including the brain, eye, and sexual organs.

One of the obstacles that precluded the more extensive use of transverse sectional anatomy was in the lack of a method which would harden the bodies or hold the parts in situ. In the early part of the last century, De Riemer, a Dutch anatomist, exhibited transverse sections of frozen bodies and later published an atlas showing, as he states, "the exact position of the internal parts of the body in relation to their mutual positions and their contact with the walls of the various cavities."

Huschke, in 1844, published ten pictures of transverse sections through the neck, thorax, abdomen, and pelvis of the cadaver of a girl 18 months old, and was so pleased by the beauty and usefulness of these sections that he said: "In case these pictures meet with favor, I shall later undertake a comprehensive study of the adult male and female body by means of transverse and longitudinal sections."

Some years later (1852–59), the great Russian anatomist and surgeon, Nicolas Pirogoff, produced a monumental work entitled *Anatome topographica, sectionibus per corpus humanum congelatum, triplici directione ductis illustrata.* This work consists of five volumes—an octavo containing 796 pages of descriptive matter and four imperial folios containing 213 plates. The first volume of plates represents life-sized sections of the head taken for the most part in transverse planes. The second volume of plates is entitled "Sectiones transversae cavi thoracis," but it also contains a number of sagittal sections. The third volume, entitled "Sectiones transversae cavi abdominis," contains a number of sagittal and frontal sections of both sexes. The fourth volume is entitled "Sectiones per extremitates et per articulos extremitatis superioris, inferiorisque triplici directione ductae."

Soon after the appearance of the first part of Pirogoff's work, Le Gendre (1858) published a work entitled "Anatomie Chirurgicale Homolographique." Published in folio, this contains 25 plates representing natural-sized sections taken in horizontal, sagittal, and oblique planes from various portions of the body. The frontispiece serves as a key figure to show the various planes of the sections. A brief text accompanies the plates. The drawings were made by the author and show little detail. Le Gendre discusses the method of enveloping the parts in gypsum employed by Weber and Arnold, the method of hardening in alcohol employed by Kohlrausch, and the method of decalcifying the entire pelvis by weak nitric acid.

Braune, in 1872, published a splendid atlas entitled "Topographisch-anatomischer Atlas. Nach Durchschnitten an gefrorenen Cadavern." The first part of Braune's atlas appeared in 1867 and contained illustrations of the sagittal sections of male and female bodies; these illustrations have since become classics. The work, containing sections taken in three planes, was completed in 1872. The text gives a very careful description of the relationships of organs and a critical discussion of the work of preceding authors. So well was the work received by the clinicians that a second edition was published in 1875, and was translated into English by E. Bellamy in 1877. Shortly after its appearance, Henke called attention to the work and emphasized the importance of making reconstructions from the sections. The third edition of Braune's atlas appeared in 1888. In the introduction to this edition, Braune refers to the suggestions made by Henke regarding reconstructions, and agrees that such would be of great value, but states that the sections must be thinner and the parts must be held in situ.

In 1873, the first part of Rüdinger's *Topographisch-chirurgische Anatomie des Menchen* appeared. The second part was published in 1874–75, the third part in 1878, and a supplemental part in 1879. The entire work contains 721 pages of text, together with 183 illustrations. There are 73 illustrations of frozen sections of the adult and newborn, taken in the three principal planes. The illustrations by photographic reproduction are excellent, but the structures are not worked out in the detail shown in Braune's atlas. In all the illustrations of sections preceding the supplemental part, the structures bear numerals that in many cases are found only after a tedious search. In the supplemental part a great improvement is made in that the structures are designated by leaders which bear numerals.

Thomas Dwight, in 1881, published a small volume entitled *Frozen Sections of a Child*. This was the first attempt in this country to emphasize the importance of studying gross anatomy by means of serial sections. The work includes an explanatory text and 25 illustrations of serial transverse section through the trunk of a three-year-old girl. Though lacking in details, his work should have stimulated other American anatomists to adopt this method of studying and teaching gross anatomy. Professor Dwight realized the importance of this method since he says: "Believing, as I do, that frozen sections will play an important part in the anatomical teaching of the future, I shall say nothing of their advantages, which speak for themselves." Symington, a few years later (1887), published a work entitled *The Topographical Anatomy of the Child,* based on a study of frozen sections and contains 14 life-sized colored plates, with a brief explanatory text.

The last attempt to produce an exhaustive work based on a study of frozen sections was made by Macewen (1893), who published an *Atlas of Head Sections*. This consists of seven series of sections: three series of coronal sections, two from an adult and one from a child; one series of sagittal sections from an adult; three series of transverse sections, two from an adult and one from a child. The text is restricted to very brief explanatory notes which accompany the sections. The work merits the distinction of being the first to show, in any detail, the skull and brain in situ. The illustrations are from copper plates made from photographs, and are as artistic as can be made from frozen sections; yet, as in all other frozen sections, the saw has destroyed or obscured many of the finer details.

The introduction of formalin as a hardening fluid marked the beginning of a new epoch in the study of sectional anatomy. It was first used by Gerota (1895), who injected a 5 percent aqueous solution of formalin, then froze and sectioned the body. A very important advance was made by Terry (1900), who injected a solution made of equal parts of 50 percent formalin and 95 percent alcohol, and obtained excellent sections without freezing. The best sections, according to Terry, are obtained from material fixed as above and then thoroughly decalcified with 10 percent hydrochloric acid.

In the following year (1901), Jackson published a method which has since been used extensively. The method is simply the thorough injection of the blood vessels with a 50 percent aqueous solution of formalin. Its points of superiority as stated by Jackson are as follows: "No freezing is necessary; the sections are made more easily and smoothly; and, finally, they do not thaw out and become loose and flabby upon handling. This method is also superior to all embedding methods, since not only the surfaces of the section, but also the structures between, are accessible for examination. In fact, it combines the advantages of dissection with those of plane sections."

The inception of the 1911 edition of *A Cross-Section Anatomy* dates back to 1902, when Dr. Eycleshymer with Dr. Dean Lewis formulated plans for a "Cross-Section Anatomy," which were approved by Dr. Lewellys F. Barker, then director of the Anatomical Laboratories of the University of Chicago. Material was being selected when it was learned that Dr. Peter Potter, of The University of Missouri, had partially completed a similar work. Subsequent events brought both Dr. Potter and Dr. Eycleshymer to St. Louis University where, during the winter of 1904, Dr. Potter completed his *Topography of the Thorax and Abdomen*. At this time, Dr. Eycleshymer suggested that the anatomical department of St. Louis University should undertake a similar but more comprehensive study. With this end in view, the task was begun. After the work on the trunk was well under way, the entire project suffered interruption when Dr. Potter and Dr. H. D. Kistler retired from the department to engage in the practice of medicine. Continuance of the work fell to Dr. Eycleshymer who later secured the cooperation of Dr. D. M. Schoemaker. Dr. Eycleshymer, Dr. Schoemaker, and Mr. Tom Jones (artist) are responsible for the original section drawings on the reconstructions of the viscera of ten subjects, which were done by Dr. Potter, and those of the female pelvis, done by Dr. Carroll Smith.

This atlas has been prepared for use by the clinician as a reference for normals when studying CT scans and echograms of the head and body, by the radiotherapist for determination of depth of organs for dosimetry planning, and by the anatomist for general reference.

Contents

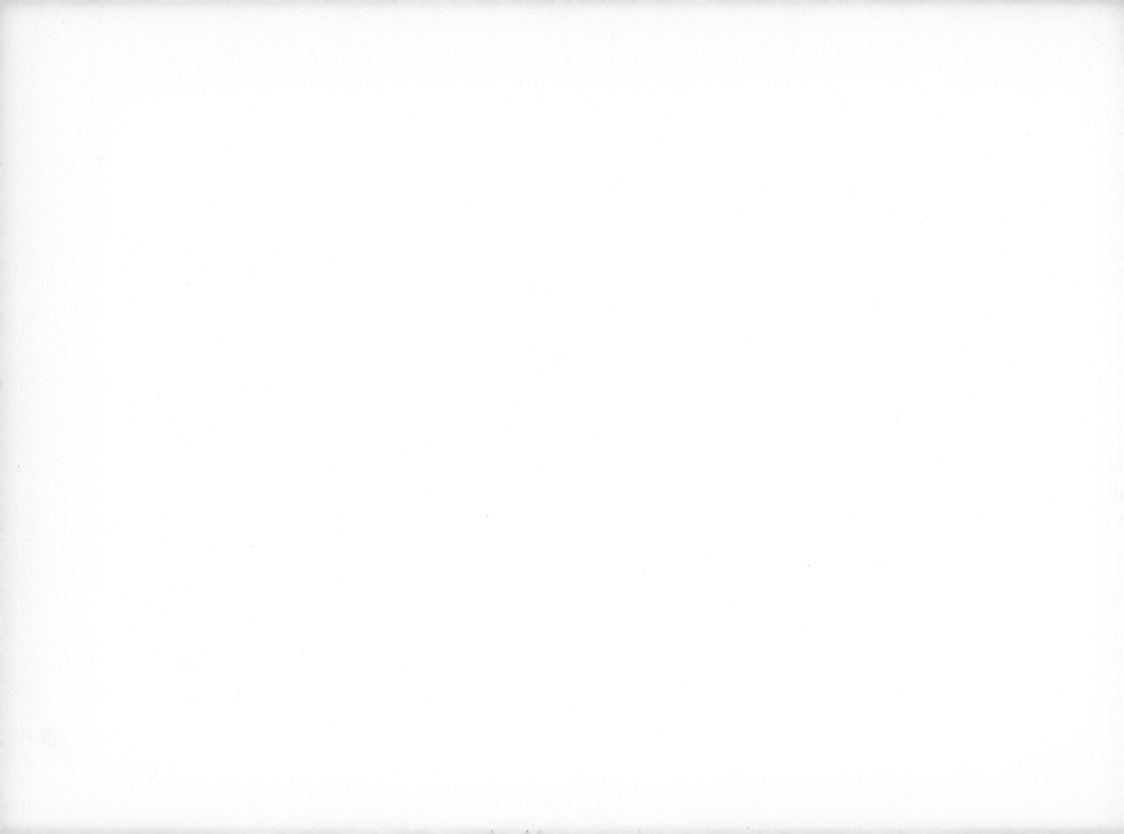

Introduction

Rapid advancement of new x-ray equipment and ultrasonography has again brought into focus the importance of a detailed knowledge of transverse cross-sectional anatomy of the human body in the current practice of medicine. Only by understanding the many variations of normal will it be possible to fully appreciate the abnormal.

Computerized tomography, introduced in 1972 by Hounsfield *, makes it possible to identify different soft tissue structures that vary by 1 to 2 percent in their absorption of x-rays. This new equipment is thus much more sensitive than x-ray film in the differentiation of various anatomic structures. The images are made in a transverse plane rather than the traditional coronal and sagittal planes.

Adapted from *A Cross-Section Anatomy* by Eycleshymer and Schoemaker, which was originally published in 1911, this atlas has been revised to correlate the images obtained by CT scanning and ultrasound with the original diagrams and with actual x-rays of human specimens. New diagrams have been drawn of the head and spine to correspond more precisely to the plane used by CT scanning. Traditionally, the anatomist has viewed the body from the head down, and the original sections were drawn accordingly. For more accurate reference, these have been miniaturized and then viewing orientation reversed to correspond directly to the CT scans and echograms. The nomenclature has been rewritten incorporating the "Nomina Anatomica" terminology approved by the Sixth International Congress of Anatomists at Paris, 1955. Medical eponyms have been used sparingly.

MATERIAL

X-rays of Specimens. The anatomic material used for x-rays throughout the atlas was prepared by placing embalmed cadavers in a Revco deep freeze unit for periods of 2 to 3 days. After freezing to a temperature of −40F, the entire body was sectioned on a band saw using section thicknesses of approximately 2 to 3 cm (joints were sectioned at approximately 0.5 cm). Following thawing to room temperature, each section was photographed and then x-rayed.

Variations in positions of organs were noted among the three bodies used. Sections were utilized which approximated the original atlas drawings as near as possible.

CT Scans and Echograms. Recent policies have been established to standardize CT scanning and ultrasound.* It has been agreed that all images should be presented as though viewing the body from the feet up (rather than from the head down). Thus all CT scans and ultrasound studies have been presented in the manner conventional for viewing x-ray films, namely; the patient's right is on the viewer's left. Since this is just the opposite for the anatomist, the larger diagram of each section has been kept as drawn, ie, viewing the body from the head down. A miniature of the diagram has also been included, reversing the right and left to correspond with the CT scan and ultrasound.

Several examples of CT scans and echograms were selected from different patients and from cadavers (scanned prior to embalming) to demonstrate variations of normal. X-rays of the sections prepared as described above have also been included and, when appearing on the following page, enlarged.

Added contrast material was used to further clarify the anatomy on the CT scan. Intravenous contrast material has been used frequently in conjunction with CT scans of the head and many times during CT scanning of the body to improve visualization of vessels, the kidneys, bladder, liver, spleen, etc. Gastrografin® has been administered to some patients to demonstrate the relative position of the gut to other structures such as the pancreas. Although some variations of normal were included, there was no attempt to cover all possibilities.

Scans through the head were obtained 30° to Reid's base line (the anthro-

* Hounsfield, GN: Computerized transverse axial scanning, Part I. Br J Radiol 46:1016–1022, 1973

* Eyler, WR, Figley, MM: Computed tomography display. Radiology 119:487–488, 1976

pologic base line), through the orbit parallel to Reid's base line, and through the body at right angles. Two new sections have been included at the end of the atlas: 1) vertical slices of the body to correspond to the longitudinal axis used by ultrasound imaging; 2) diagrams and transverse scans of the normal spine selected to serve as a reference, since the spine is seen in cross-section on all CT scans of the body. Two anatomic drawings are provided with each vertebral body scan. One is a representation of the CT scan, depicting the slice in the vertebral column. The other is an axial view of the disarticulated vertebral body to demonstrate the surface anatomy.

PROCEDURES

Computed Tomography. The computed tomographic (CT) scanner is an x-ray machine capable of producing a cross-sectional image on a television monitor. Mathematical formulas are used to calculate very slight differences in the absorption coefficients of different tissue to an x-ray beam which passes through the body from a number of directions around or parallel to the transverse axis. The large number of equations involved requires the use of a computer, and many modifications have been made to refine this technique so that an image can now be obtained with greater detail in less time.

The images for this atlas were made using an Ohio-Nuclear Delta Whole-Body Scanner with a 13 mm collimator. The patient is placed on a table top equipped with a belt which moves automatically at 2.6 cm increments through the plane of the x-ray beam. The actual distance that the patient moves between the paired sections may be varied according to the area under study, allowing for considerable overlap or for widely separated sections. An x-ray tube with two finely collimated and filtered beams, each 1.3 cm in diameter, is centered precisely over a group of calcium fluoride detectors (three for each x-ray beam). The x-ray tube and detectors are mounted on a yoke, traverse the plane of the patient, rotate 3° parallel to the transverse plane of the patient, then repeat the traverse. This movement is continued throughout 180° for a total of 60 traverses, completing the scan within 2.5 minutes for the whole body.

During each traverse, over 30,000 individual readings of the absorbed x-ray beam are recorded by the detectors as quanta of x-ray transmission and processed in preparation for entry into the computer, which reconstructs the image on a 256 x 256 matrix format (or 65,536 picture elements).

This requires high-speed computational circuits to solve over 65,536 mathematical equations by a section known as the "convolver." The final summation of picture elements or "pixels" are stored temporarily on a disc, then transferred to a magnetic tape for permanent storage. The images are reproduced for viewing on a television monitor as they are formed and are recorded on film for the patient's records.

Very fine differences in tissue absorption of 1 to 1.5 percent result in the identification of tumor, edema, infarction, etc., within the brain substance and in the separation of gray and white matter of brain. A gray scale has been used which is directly related to the absorption coefficients of tissue (calculated by formula *) and ranges from −1,000 units for the minimum absorption of air (black) to +1,000 for the maximum absorption of dense bone (white), with water being equal to zero. The contrast and density of the image projected on the TV monitor can be varied by the viewer using the controls provided. A broad spectrum encompassing a variety of the tissues in the image may be seen by using a wide window that cover the entire gray scale but has poor contrast. A narrow window results in a shortened spectrum with good contrast. The centering of this window is varied for the tissue of interest, eg, −150 to −400 for the lung, +150 to +300 for bone, +40 for kidney, etc. The individual figures are expressed as Delta units.

Each year, new generations of machines have evolved rapidly with improved equipment and simplified computation. The prototype of the EMI™ head unit required a water bag around the head, took 4½ minutes for each scan, and used an 80 x 80 matrix. The longer scan times produced problems with motion artifacts, ie, areas of high and low absorption units (white and black lines) recorded on the image caused by the movement of any object of high contrast (metallic clips, air within the gut) during the scan. Movement may be due to peristalsis, respiration, or an uncooperative patient. With the newer equipment, a scan can now be completed in 5 to 20 seconds and the image convolved immediately. New detectors with improved software providing even faster timing and better resolution are in the process of evaluation. The CT scanning illustrations in this atlas represent the state of the art as it now exists (1975–1976).

Ultrasound. Ultrasonic cross-sections are produced by mapping echoes produced by high-frequency sound waves transmitted into the body. These echoes are reflected at interfaces where there is a change in acoustic properties, ie, in

* Hounsfield, GN: Picture quality of computed tomography. Am J Radiol 127:3–9, 1976

density or sound velocity. The sound waves are generated by means of a piezo-electric crystal which is placed in close contact with the skin, usually with an oil or a gel coupling medium. The crystal acts both as a transmitter and as a receiver. In the transmission phase, a short pulse of ultrasound (typically 1 to 5 MHz) is generated. The crystal then acts as a receiver for the returning echo. Since the velocity of sound in most tissues and fluids in the body is reasonably uniform (about 1500m/sec), it is possible to compute the distance of the echo from the transducer. This is done by means of a cathode-ray tube, which displays both the starting point of the signal (at the transducer) as well as the location of the echo on an oscilloscope screen.

The position of the transducer is controlled by an arm which is connected to potentiometers that change the positional signal into an electrical one. This electrical signal is also fed into the cathode-ray tube and results in the beam on the oscilloscope screen moving in direct relation to the motion of the transducer.

The beam shape of the ultrasound signal produced by the transducer is a critical factor in determining the lateral resolution of the system. The beam tends to widen at increasing distance from the transducer, with consequent resolution loss. This can be modified somewhat through the use of various ultrasonic collimating lens systems. The depth resolution is determined by the length of the pulse and the frequency of the sound waves. In the illustrations used in this atlas, depth resolution is within 1 to 2 mm and lateral resolution within 1.2 cm.

While soft tissues, such as muscle and most parenchymal organs, transmit sound quite well, it is not possible to obtain echoes through bone or air-containing structures. Bony structures reflect sound strongly from their closest surface, and a shadow is produced beyond this interface from which no information can be obtained. Air-containing structures attenuate sound very rapidly. Thus a shadow is also produced beyond an air-containing structure from which no echoes are recordable.

The problems with poor lateral resolution, as well as loss of echoes due to intervening bone or air-containing structures, are partly overcome by the use of a compound scanning technique. In this technique, the transducer is gently rotated back and forth as it is moved over the surface of the body, thus providing multiple opportunities for obtaining each possible echo. This allows the surfaces of bone or air-containing structures to be seen from the side. The use of compounding also permits sharper depth resolution, which partly offsets the poor lateral resolution.

While the strength of the echo is largely determined by the acoustical properties of the structures at the interface, it depends upon the physical dimensions and direction of this interface. Basically, echoes follow the same laws of reflection as light waves and will therefore be most strongly seen when a surface is perpendicular to the echo beam. These are known as specular reflections, and their intensity is very strongly dependent upon the direction of the ultrasound beam. In addition, echoes are produced at smaller surfaces, eg, at the interface between muscle bundles. Such relatively irregular surfaces produce echoes that are much softer and less spatially directed. These are known as diffuse echoes. Recent progress in ultrasound technology allows for a display of both specular and diffuse echoes by instruments known as "grey scale" ultrasound scanners.

Each of the ultrasonic sections illustrated in the atlas took approximately 30 to 60 seconds to complete. As a result, there is some loss of resolution due to motion. There is also loss due to the mechanical-electrical linkage system sensing the transducer position, which can at best be adjusted to an accuracy of about 3 mm. The manual transducer motion, along with the variability of specular reflections, assures that no two echograms obtained under similar circumstances will ever appear identical.

The major clinical applications of the ultrasound technique illustrated in this atlas are in the diagnosis of lesions of the thyroid, liver, pancreas, kidney, retroperitoneum, and pelvis. A particularly important use of ultrasound is with respect to the gravid uterus, where it is helpful not only because of the abundance of soft-tissue structures that can be differentiated, but also because the ultrasonic radiation is nonionizing and is not known to cause any biologic hazard.

Ultrasonic cross-sections can be obtained in any direction. Transverse and vertical sections are inspected from below, and vertical sections with the head to the left. In clinical work, an orientation system based on some easily palpable physical landmarks, such as the iliac crest or sternal notch, is usually employed to identify the position of cross-section. In the preparation of cross-sections for this atlas, an effort was made to match them as closely as possible to the anatomic drawings. Ultrasound sections were omitted in areas such as the head and thorax, where only limited information is obtainable on ultrasonic echography.

CROSS-SECTIONAL ANATOMY

Computed Tomography
and
Ultrasound Correlation

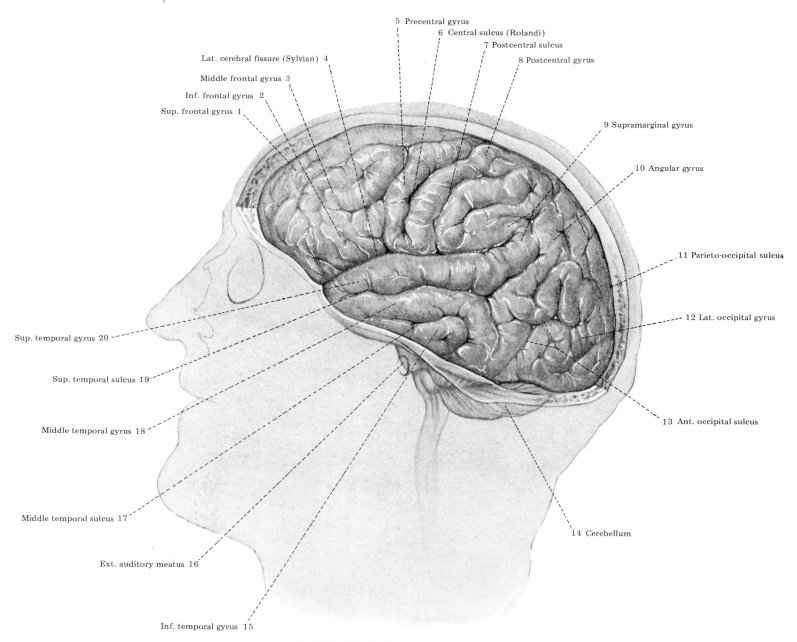

5 Precentral gyrus

6 Central sulcus (Rolandi)

7 Postcentral sulcus

8 Postcentral gyrus

Lat. cerebral fissure (Sylvian) 4

Middle frontal gyrus 3

Inf. frontal gyrus 2

Sup. frontal gyrus 1

9 Supramarginal gyrus

10 Angular gyrus

11 Parieto-occipital sulcus

12 Lat. occipital gyrus

Sup. temporal gyrus 20

13 Ant. occipital sulcus

Sup. temporal sulcus 19

Middle temporal gyrus 18

14 Cerebellum

Middle temporal sulcus 17

Ext. auditory meatus 16

Inf. temporal gyrus 15

KEY FIGURE I Lateral surface of brain.

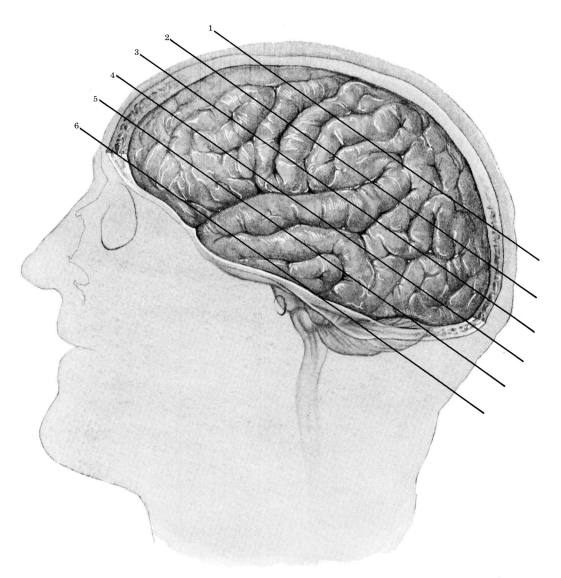

KEY FIGURE II Reference levels taken at 30° to the anthropologic baseline superimposed on the lateral surface of the brain.

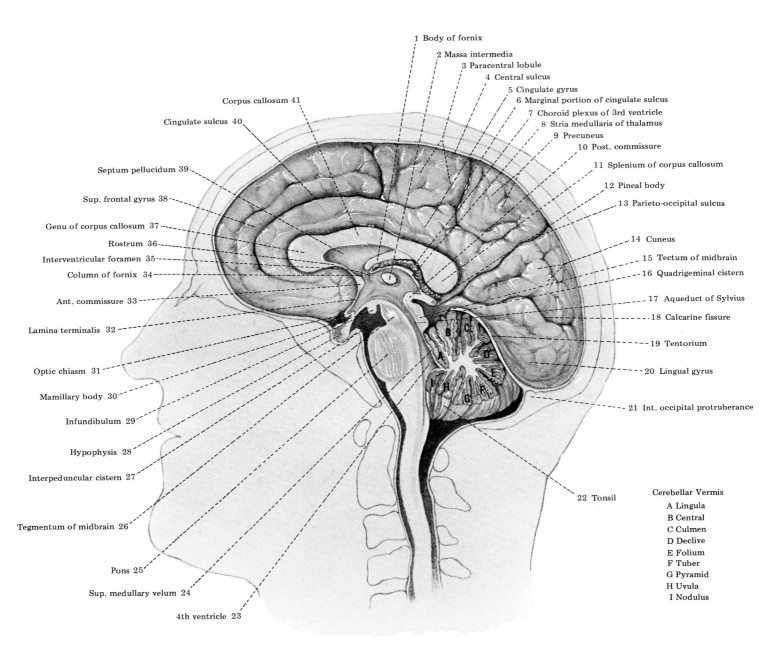

1 Body of fornix
2 Massa intermedia
3 Paracentral lobule
4 Central sulcus
5 Cingulate gyrus
6 Marginal portion of cingulate sulcus
7 Choroid plexus of 3rd ventricle
8 Stria medullaris of thalamus
9 Precuneus
10 Post. commissure
11 Splenium of corpus callosum
12 Pineal body
13 Parieto-occipital sulcus
14 Cuneus
15 Tectum of midbrain
16 Quadrigeminal cistern
17 Aqueduct of Sylvius
18 Calcarine fissure
19 Tentorium
20 Lingual gyrus
21 Int. occipital protruberance
22 Tonsil

Corpus callosum 41
Cingulate sulcus 40
Septum pellucidum 39
Sup. frontal gyrus 38
Genu of corpus callosum 37
Rostrum 36
Interventricular foramen 35
Column of fornix 34
Ant. commissure 33
Lamina terminalis 32
Optic chiasm 31
Mamillary body 30
Infundibulum 29
Hypophysis 28
Interpeduncular cistern 27
Tegmentum of midbrain 26
Pons 25
Sup. medullary velum 24
4th ventricle 23

Cerebellar Vermis
A Lingula
B Central
C Culmen
D Declive
E Folium
F Tuber
G Pyramid
H Uvula
I Nodulus

KEY FIGURE III   Midline sagittal section of brain.

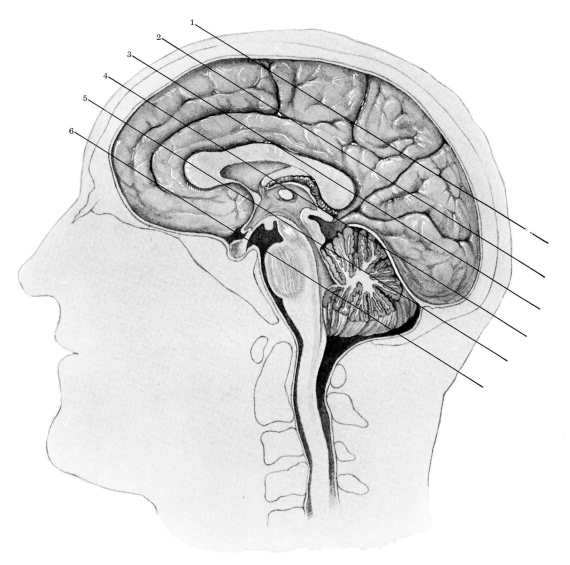

KEY FIGURE IV Reference levels taken at 30° to the anthropologic baseline superimposed on midline sagittal section.

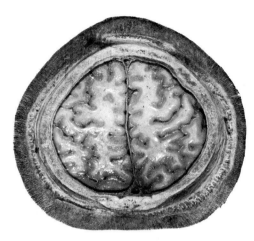

Section 1 (specimen)

Cingulate gyrus 21

1 Sup. sagittal sinus

2 Sup. frontal gyrus

Middle frontal gyrus 20

3 Falx cerebri

4 Dura mater

Precentral sulcus 19

5 Precentral sulcus

Precentral gyrus 18

6 Central sulcus

Central sulcus 17

7 Postcentral gyrus

Sup. parietal lobe 16

8 Subarachnoid space

Precuneus 15

Skin 14

Subcutaneous connective tissue 13

9 Longitudinal cerebral fissure

Galea aponeurotica 12

11 Skull

10 Sup. sagittal sinus

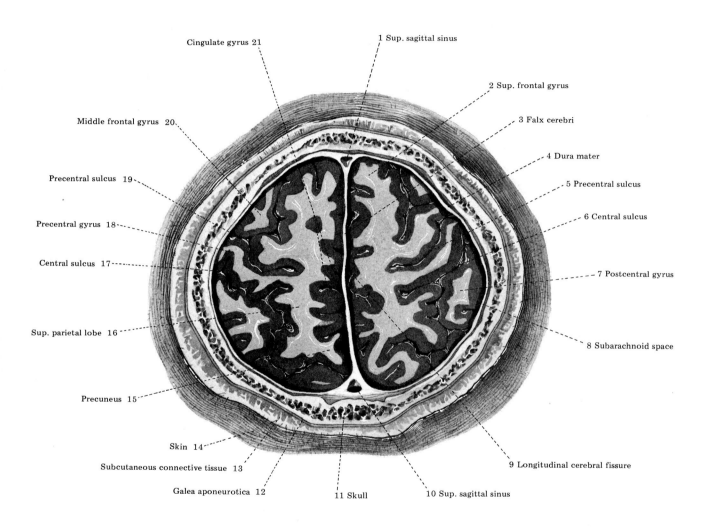

Section 1

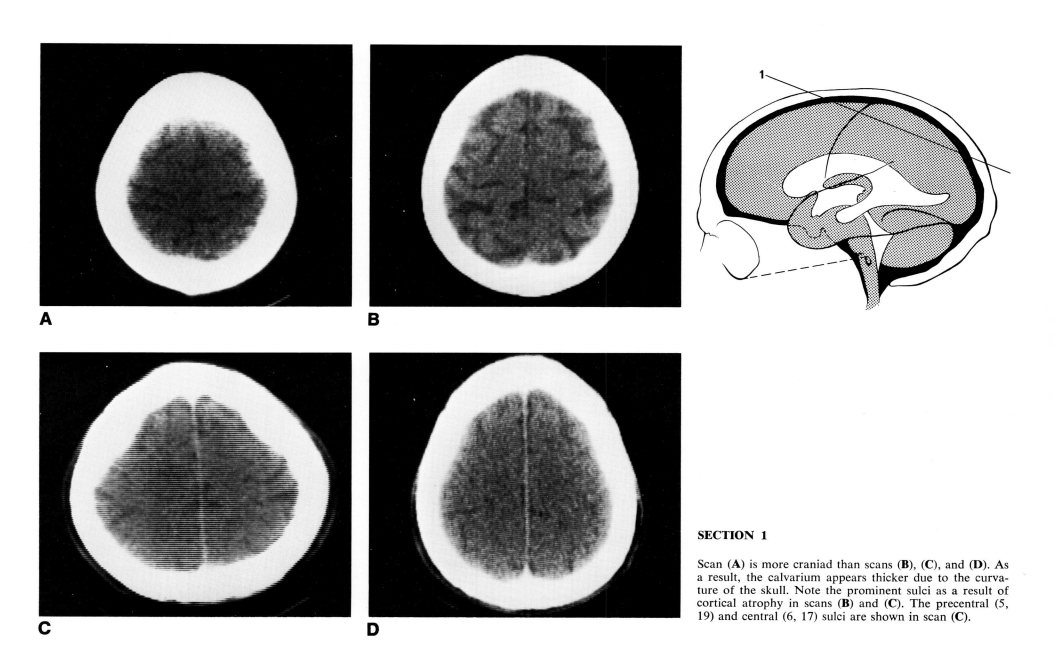

A

B

C

D

1

SECTION 1

Scan (**A**) is more craniad than scans (**B**), (**C**), and (**D**). As a result, the calvarium appears thicker due to the curvature of the skull. Note the prominent sulci as a result of cortical atrophy in scans (**B**) and (**C**). The precentral (5, 19) and central (6, 17) sulci are shown in scan (**C**).

Section 1

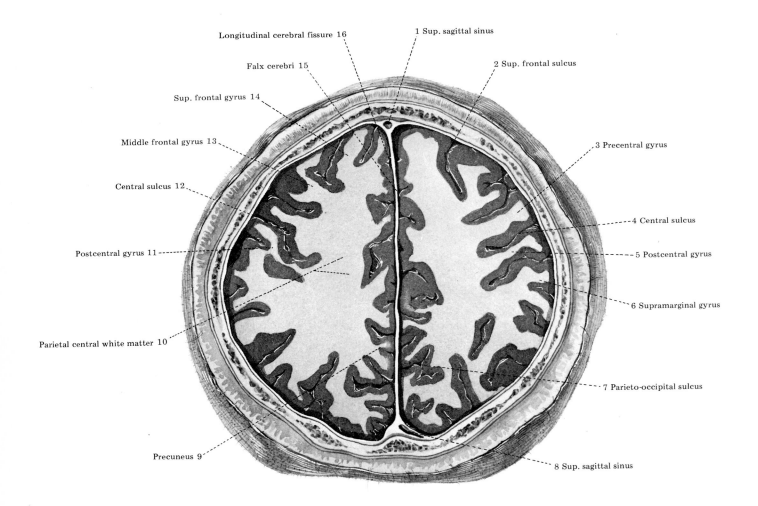

Longitudinal cerebral fissure 16

1 Sup. sagittal sinus

Falx cerebri 15

2 Sup. frontal sulcus

Sup. frontal gyrus 14

Middle frontal gyrus 13

3 Precentral gyrus

Central sulcus 12

4 Central sulcus

Postcentral gyrus 11

5 Postcentral gyrus

6 Supramarginal gyrus

Parietal central white matter 10

7 Parieto-occipital sulcus

Precuneus 9

8 Sup. sagittal sinus

Section 2 (specimen)

Section 2

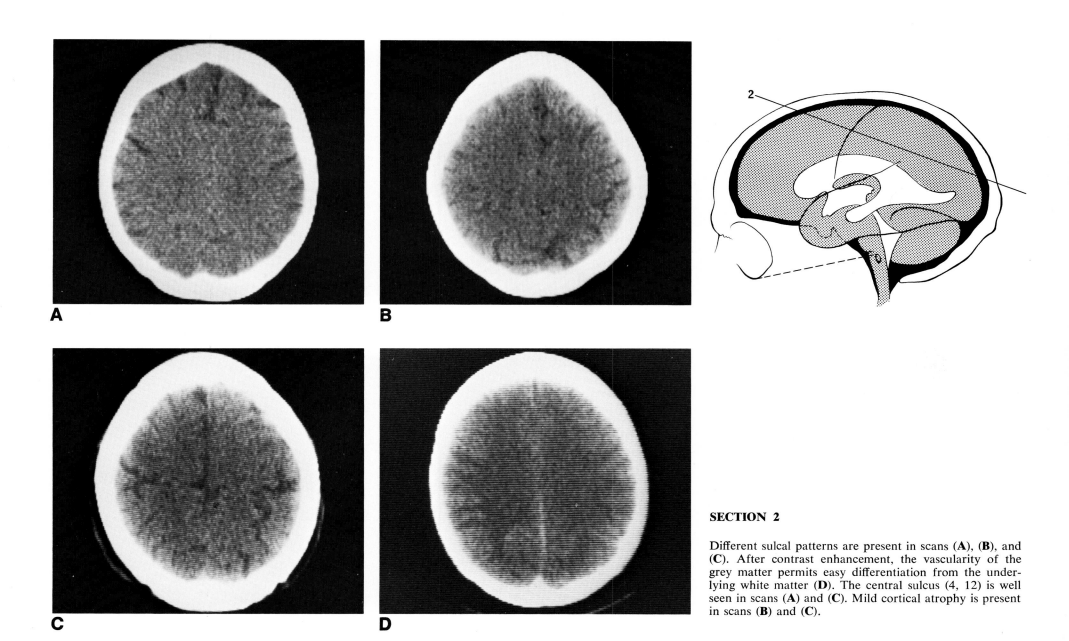

A

B

C

D

2

SECTION 2

Different sulcal patterns are present in scans (**A**), (**B**), and (**C**). After contrast enhancement, the vascularity of the grey matter permits easy differentiation from the underlying white matter (**D**). The central sulcus (4, 12) is well seen in scans (**A**) and (**C**). Mild cortical atrophy is present in scans (**B**) and (**C**).

Section 2

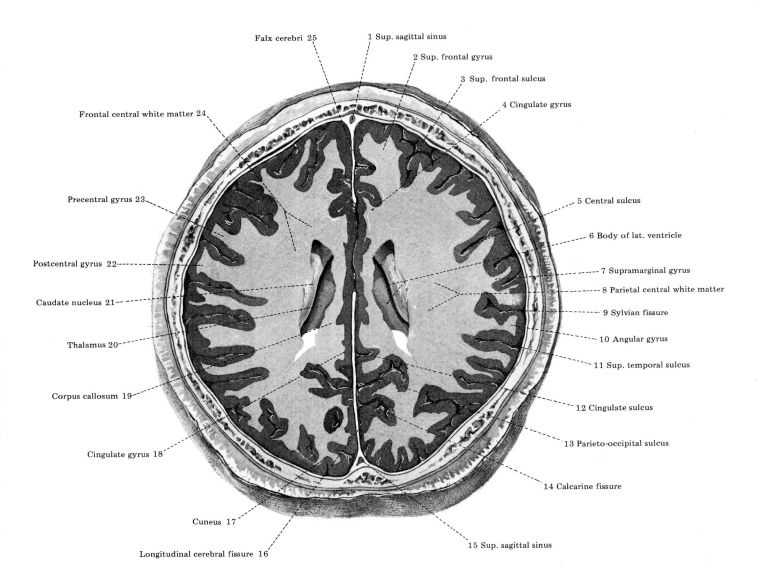

Falx cerebri 25

1 Sup. sagittal sinus

2 Sup. frontal gyrus

3 Sup. frontal sulcus

4 Cingulate gyrus

Frontal central white matter 24

5 Central sulcus

6 Body of lat. ventricle

Precentral gyrus 23

7 Supramarginal gyrus

8 Parietal central white matter

Postcentral gyrus 22

9 Sylvian fissure

Caudate nucleus 21

10 Angular gyrus

Thalamus 20

11 Sup. temporal sulcus

12 Cingulate sulcus

Corpus callosum 19

13 Parieto-occipital sulcus

Cingulate gyrus 18

14 Calcarine fissure

Cuneus 17

15 Sup. sagittal sinus

Longitudinal cerebral fissure 16

Section 3

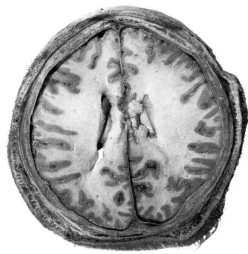

Section 3 (specimen)

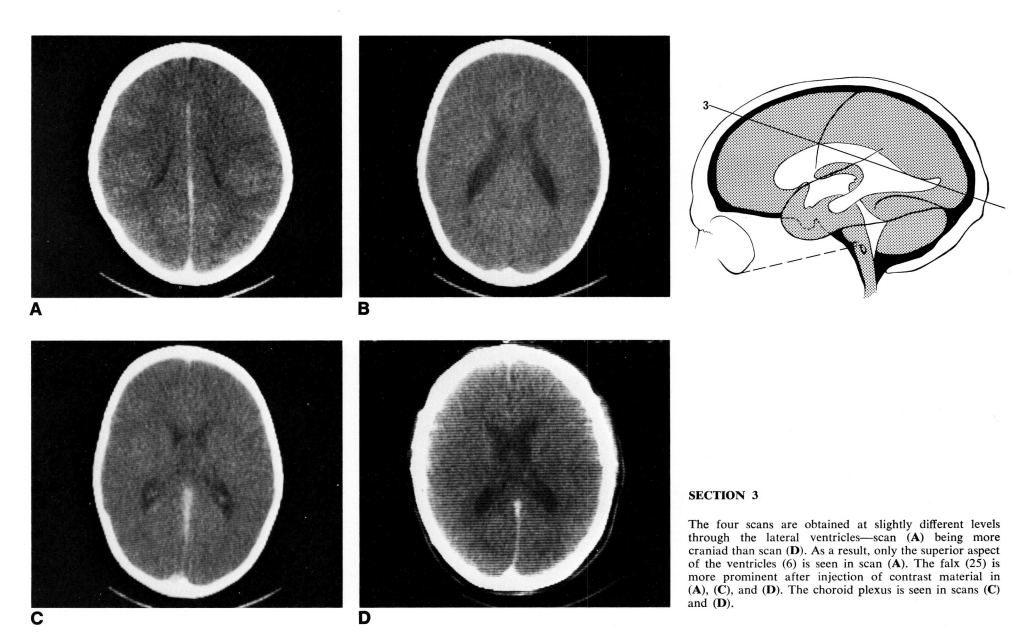

A

B

C

D

SECTION 3

The four scans are obtained at slightly different levels through the lateral ventricles—scan (**A**) being more craniad than scan (**D**). As a result, only the superior aspect of the ventricles (6) is seen in scan (**A**). The falx (25) is more prominent after injection of contrast material in (**A**), (**C**), and (**D**). The choroid plexus is seen in scans (**C**) and (**D**).

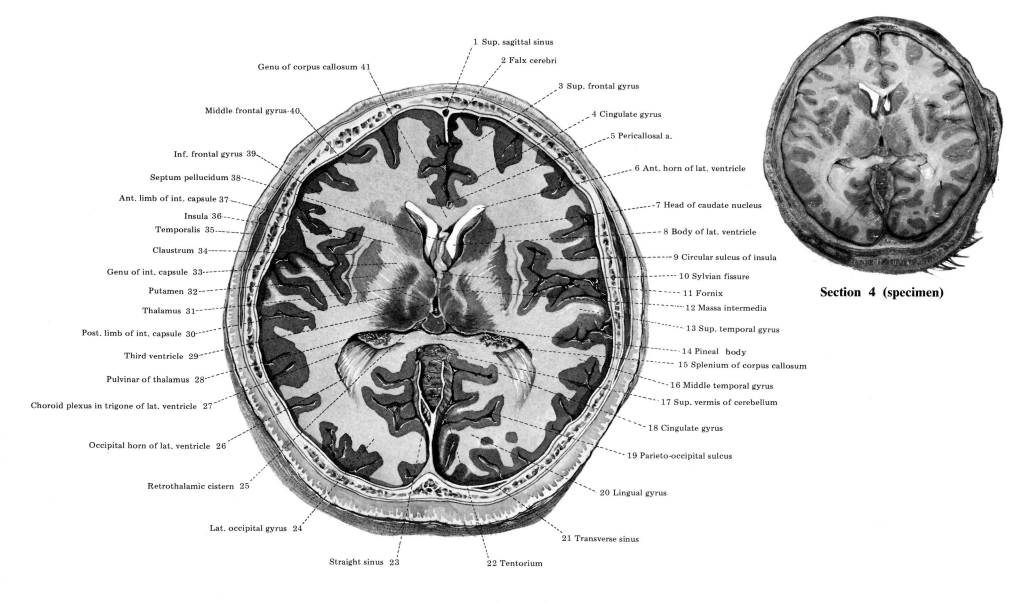

1 Sup. sagittal sinus

2 Falx cerebri

Genu of corpus callosum 41

3 Sup. frontal gyrus

Middle frontal gyrus 40

4 Cingulate gyrus

5 Pericallosal a.

Inf. frontal gyrus 39

6 Ant. horn of lat. ventricle

Septum pellucidum 38

7 Head of caudate nucleus

Ant. limb of int. capsule 37

Insula 36

8 Body of lat. ventricle

Temporalis 35

9 Circular sulcus of insula

Claustrum 34

10 Sylvian fissure

Genu of int. capsule 33

11 Fornix

Putamen 32

12 Massa intermedia

Thalamus 31

13 Sup. temporal gyrus

Post. limb of int. capsule 30

14 Pineal body

Third ventricle 29

15 Splenium of corpus callosum

Pulvinar of thalamus 28

16 Middle temporal gyrus

Choroid plexus in trigone of lat. ventricle 27

17 Sup. vermis of cerebellum

18 Cingulate gyrus

Occipital horn of lat. ventricle 26

19 Parieto-occipital sulcus

Retrothalamic cistern 25

20 Lingual gyrus

Lat. occipital gyrus 24

21 Transverse sinus

Straight sinus 23

22 Tentorium

Section 4 (specimen)

Section 4

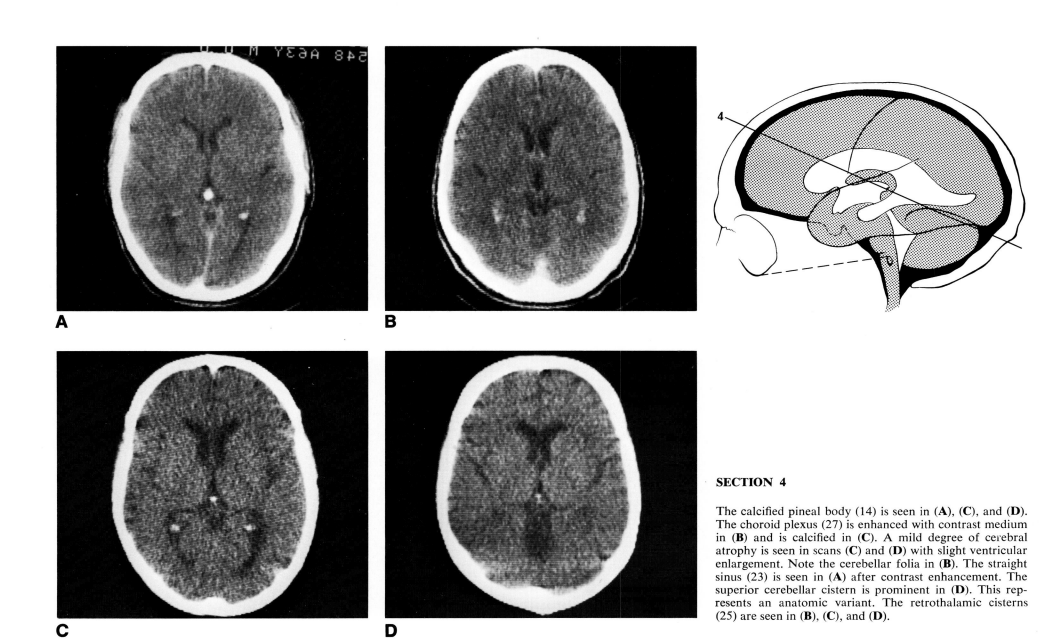

SECTION 4

The calcified pineal body (14) is seen in (**A**), (**C**), and (**D**). The choroid plexus (27) is enhanced with contrast medium in (**B**) and is calcified in (**C**). A mild degree of cerebral atrophy is seen in scans (**C**) and (**D**) with slight ventricular enlargement. Note the cerebellar folia in (**B**). The straight sinus (23) is seen in (**A**) after contrast enhancement. The superior cerebellar cistern is prominent in (**D**). This represents an anatomic variant. The retrothalamic cisterns (25) are seen in (**B**), (**C**), and (**D**).

A

B

C

D

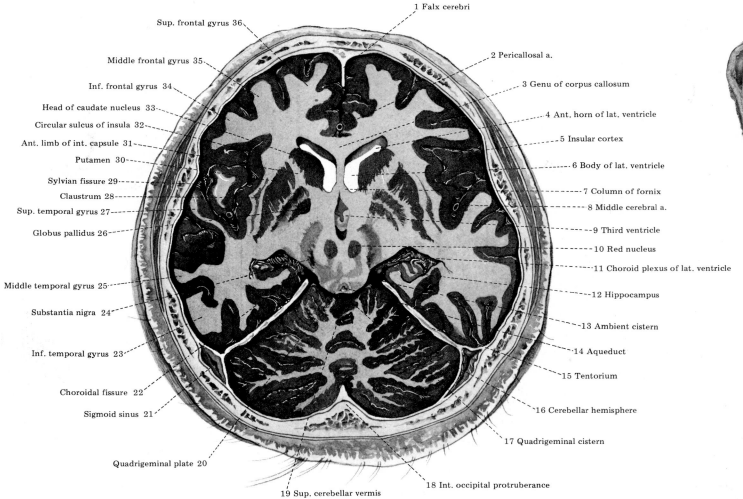

1 Falx cerebri

Sup. frontal gyrus 36

Middle frontal gyrus 35

Inf. frontal gyrus 34

Head of caudate nucleus 33

Circular sulcus of insula 32

Ant. limb of int. capsule 31

Putamen 30

Sylvian fissure 29

Claustrum 28

Sup. temporal gyrus 27

Globus pallidus 26

Middle temporal gyrus 25

Substantia nigra 24

Inf. temporal gyrus 23

Choroidal fissure 22

Sigmoid sinus 21

Quadrigeminal plate 20

19 Sup. cerebellar vermis

2 Pericallosal a.

3 Genu of corpus callosum

4 Ant. horn of lat. ventricle

5 Insular cortex

6 Body of lat. ventricle

7 Column of fornix

8 Middle cerebral a.

9 Third ventricle

10 Red nucleus

11 Choroid plexus of lat. ventricle

12 Hippocampus

13 Ambient cistern

14 Aqueduct

15 Tentorium

16 Cerebellar hemisphere

17 Quadrigeminal cistern

18 Int. occipital protruberance

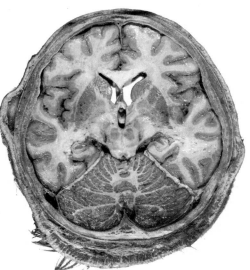

Section 5 (specimen)

Section 5

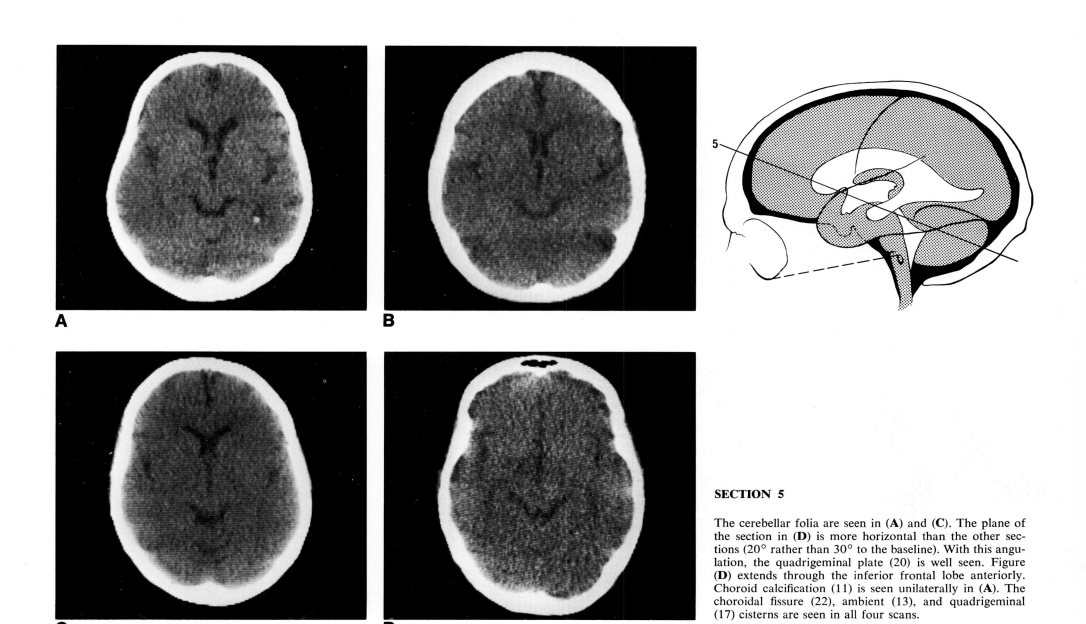

A

B

C

D

SECTION 5

The cerebellar folia are seen in (**A**) and (**C**). The plane of
the section in (**D**) is more horizontal than the other sections (20° rather than 30° to the baseline). With this angu-
lation, the quadrigeminal plate (20) is well seen. Figure
(**D**) extends through the inferior frontal lobe anteriorly.
Choroid calcification (11) is seen unilaterally in (**A**). The
choroidal fissure (22), ambient (13), and quadrigeminal
(17) cisterns are seen in all four scans.

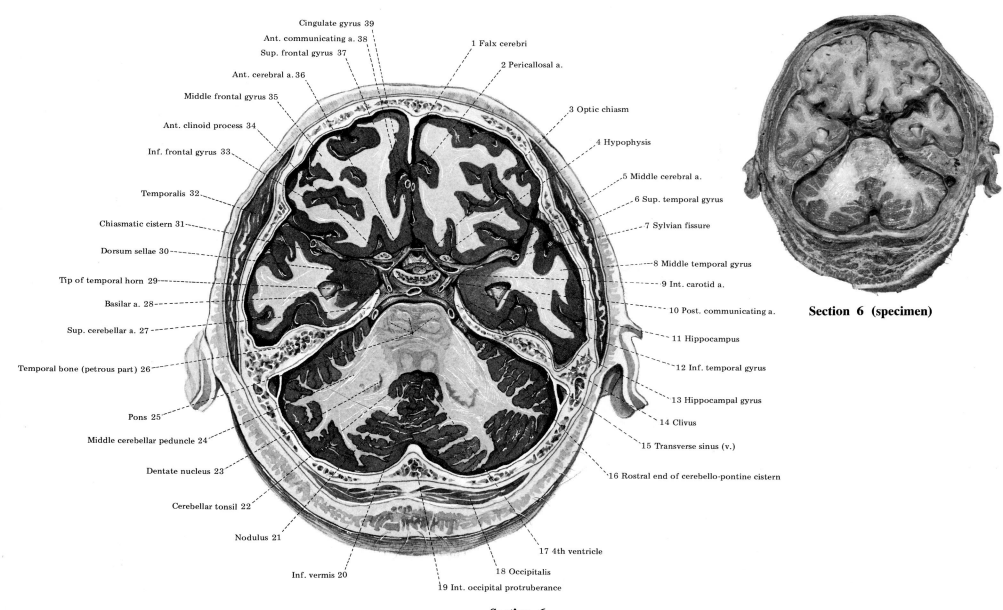

Cingulate gyrus 39

Ant. communicating a. 38

Sup. frontal gyrus 37

Ant. cerebral a. 36

Middle frontal gyrus 35

Ant. clinoid process 34

Inf. frontal gyrus 33

Temporalis 32

Chiasmatic cistern 31

Dorsum sellae 30

Tip of temporal horn 29

Basilar a. 28

Sup. cerebellar a. 27

Temporal bone (petrous part) 26

Pons 25

Middle cerebellar peduncle 24

Dentate nucleus 23

Cerebellar tonsil 22

Nodulus 21

Inf. vermis 20

19 Int. occipital protruberance

1 Falx cerebri

2 Pericallosal a.

3 Optic chiasm

4 Hypophysis

5 Middle cerebral a.

6 Sup. temporal gyrus

7 Sylvian fissure

8 Middle temporal gyrus

9 Int. carotid a.

10 Post. communicating a.

11 Hippocampus

12 Inf. temporal gyrus

13 Hippocampal gyrus

14 Clivus

15 Transverse sinus (v.)

16 Rostral end of cerebello-pontine cistern

17 4th ventricle

18 Occipitalis

Section 6 (specimen)

Section 6

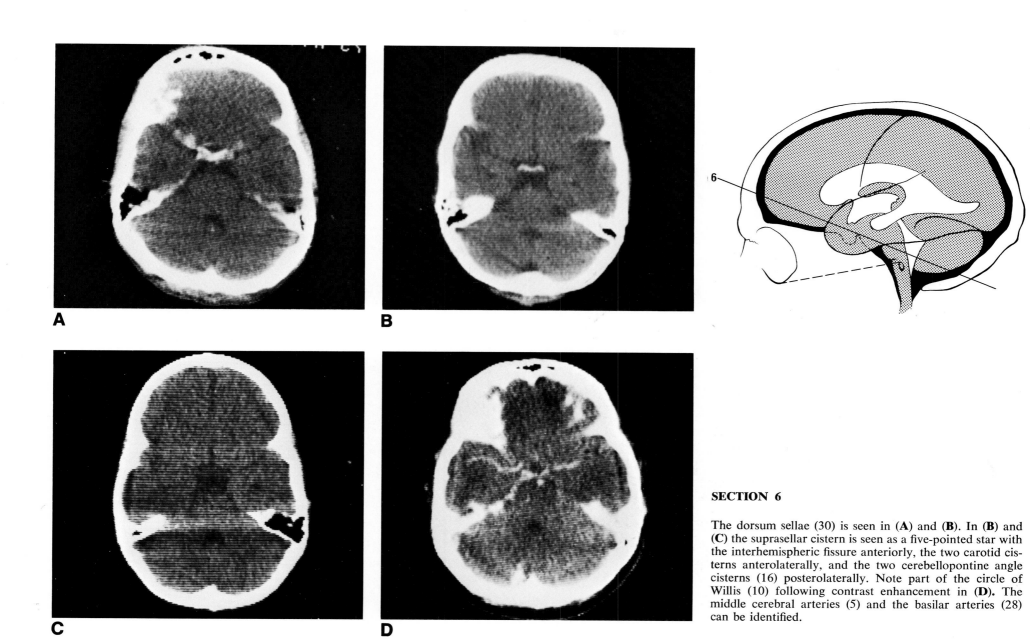

A

B

C

D

SECTION 6

The dorsum sellae (30) is seen in (**A**) and (**B**). In (**B**) and (**C**) the suprasellar cistern is seen as a five-pointed star with the interhemispheric fissure anteriorly, the two carotid cisterns anterolaterally, and the two cerebellopontine angle cisterns (16) posterolaterally. Note part of the circle of Willis (10) following contrast enhancement in (**D**). The middle cerebral arteries (5) and the basilar arteries (28) can be identified.

Section 6

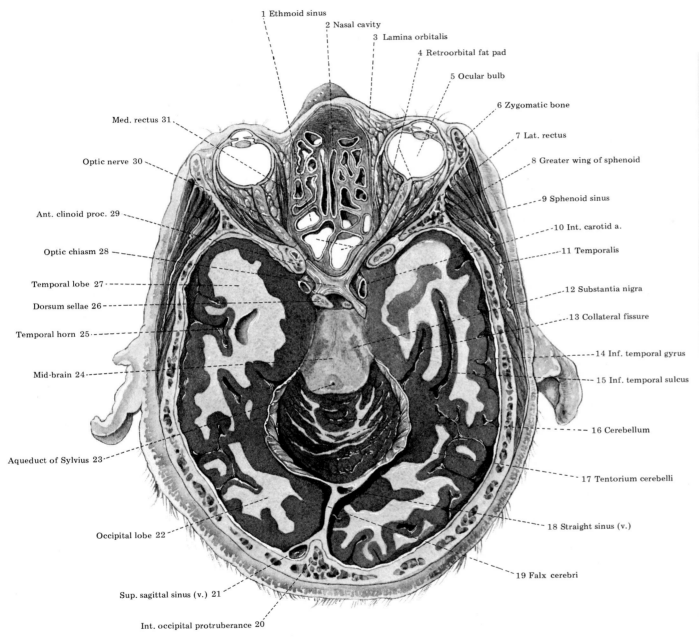

1 Ethmoid sinus
2 Nasal cavity
3 Lamina orbitalis
4 Retroorbital fat pad
5 Ocular bulb
6 Zygomatic bone
7 Lat. rectus
8 Greater wing of sphenoid
9 Sphenoid sinus
10 Int. carotid a.
11 Temporalis
12 Substantia nigra
13 Collateral fissure
14 Inf. temporal gyrus
15 Inf. temporal sulcus
16 Cerebellum
17 Tentorium cerebelli
18 Straight sinus (v.)
19 Falx cerebri

Med. rectus 31
Optic nerve 30
Ant. clinoid proc. 29
Optic chiasm 28
Temporal lobe 27
Dorsum sellae 26
Temporal horn 25
Mid-brain 24
Aqueduct of Sylvius 23
Occipital lobe 22
Sup. sagittal sinus (v.) 21
Int. occipital protruberance 20

Section 7

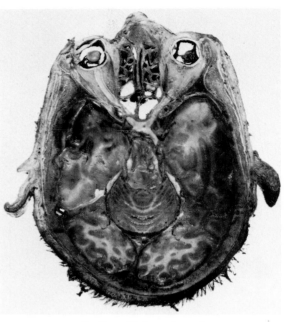

Section 7 (specimen)

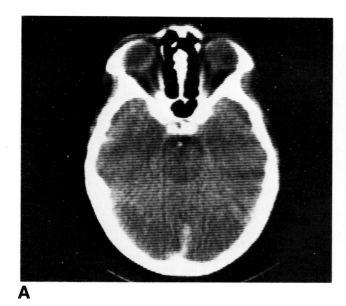

A

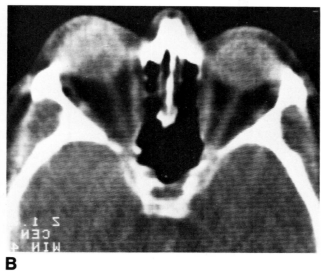

B

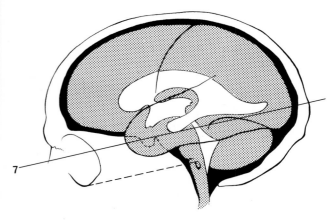

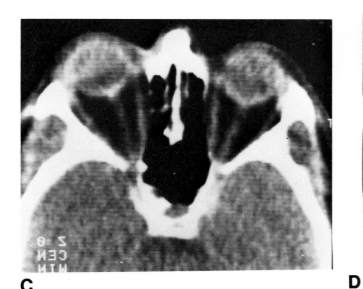

C

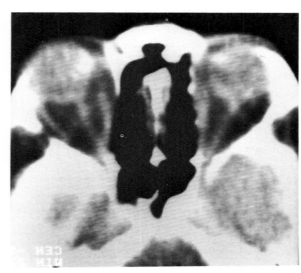

D

SECTION 7

Orbital scans are taken parallel to the anthropologic baseline as seen in (**A**). Figures (**B**), (**C**), and (**D**) represent enlargements of the orbits. Note the definition of the optic nerves (30) as well as the medial (31) and lateral (7) recti muscles in (**B**) and (**C**). Figure (**D**) is taken at a slightly craniad level through the upper quadrant of the orbit. The linear densities extending from the median walls of the orbits posterolaterally represent the superior ophthalmic veins.

NASAL CAVITY 97
Nasal bone 96
ETHMOID BONE (perpendicular plate) 95
MAXILLA (frontal proc.) 94
NASAL CAVITY 93
Quadratus labii superioris 92
Nasolacrimal duct 91
LACRIMAL BONE 90
Nose (middle & sup. meatus) 89
NASAL CAVITY 88
Ethmoidal sinuses 87
Inf. tarsus & hypophysis 86
Eye (ant. chamber) & vitreous body 85
Inf. rectus & ethmoidal sinuses 84
Oculomotor n. (inf. br.) 83
Sup. ophthalmic v. 82
Orbicularis oculi 81
Inf. oblique & lat. rectus 80
Ophthalmic n. 79
ZYGOMATIC BONE (frontosphenoidal proc.) 78
Int. carotid a. 77
Temporal pole 76
Inf. petrosal sinus (v.) 75
Abducens n. 74
Sup. temporal gyrus 73
Temporalis fascia 72
Temporalis 71
Pons (superficial transverse fibers) 70
TEMPORAL BONE 69
Hippocampal gyrus 68
Middle temporal v. 67
Middle temporal gyrus 66
Superficial temporal a. 65
Pons (deep transverse fibers) 64
Ant. auricular 63
Trigeminal n. 62
Sup. auricular 61
Facial n. 60
Acoustic n. 59
TEMPORAL BONE 58
Pons (superficial transverse fibers) 57
Inf. temporal gyrus 56
Flocculus 55
Occipitalis & transverse sinus (v.) 54
Fusiform gyrus 53
Brachium pontis 52
Sup. semilunar lobule 51
Lingual gyrus 50
Sup. cerebellar peduncle 49
Lat. occipital gyrus 48
Ant. medullary velum 47
Declive 46

1 Procerus
2 Middle nasal concha
3 MAXILLA (frontal proc.)
4 Quadratus labii sup.
5 Nasolacrimal duct
6 Bulla ethmoidalis
7 Maxilla (orbital plate)
8 Inf. oblique
9 Sphenoid bone (body)
10 MAXILLARY SINUS
11 Inf. rectus
12 Pterygopalatine fossa
13 Oculomotor n. (inf. br.)
14 Sup. & inf. orbital fissures
15 Orbicularis oculi
16 Zygomatic bone (orbital plate)
17 INT. CAROTID a.
18 Zygomatic bone (frontosphenoidal proc.)
19 Lat. pterygoid
20 Semilunar ganglion (Gasserian)
21 Middle meningeal a.
22 Temporalis
23 Trigeminal n. (motor br.)
24 Basilar a. & inf. petrosal sinus
25 Temporalis fascia
26 TEMPORAL BONE
27 Inf. temporal gyrus
28 Superficial temporal a. & v. & auriculotemporal n.
29 Greater superficial petrosal n.
30 Temporal bone (petrous portion) & cochlea
31 Epitympanic recess & malleus (head)
32 Facial n.
33 Acoustic n. & sup. semicircular canal
34 Tympanic antrum & post. auricular
35 TEMPORAL BONE (mastoid proc.)
36 Ant. inf. cerebellar a. & transverse sinus (v.)
37 Longitudinal fasciculi
38 Brachium pontis
39 Sup. semilunar lobule
40 Transverse sinus (v.)
41 Sup. cerebellar peduncle
42 Occipitalis
43 4th ventricle
44 Nodulus & INT. OCCIPITAL PROTRUBERANCE
45 Straight sinus & transverse sinus (v.)

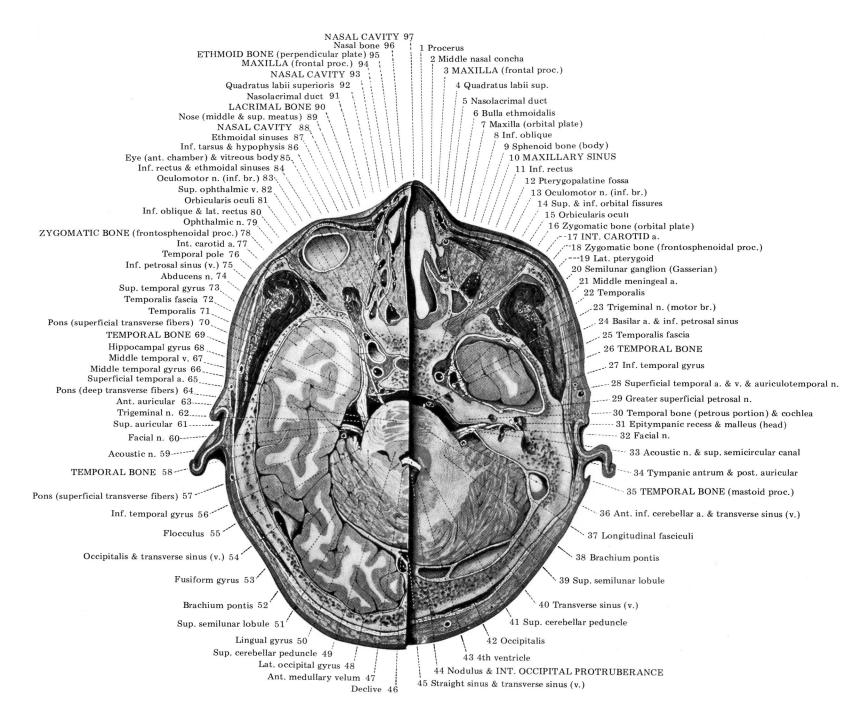

Section 8

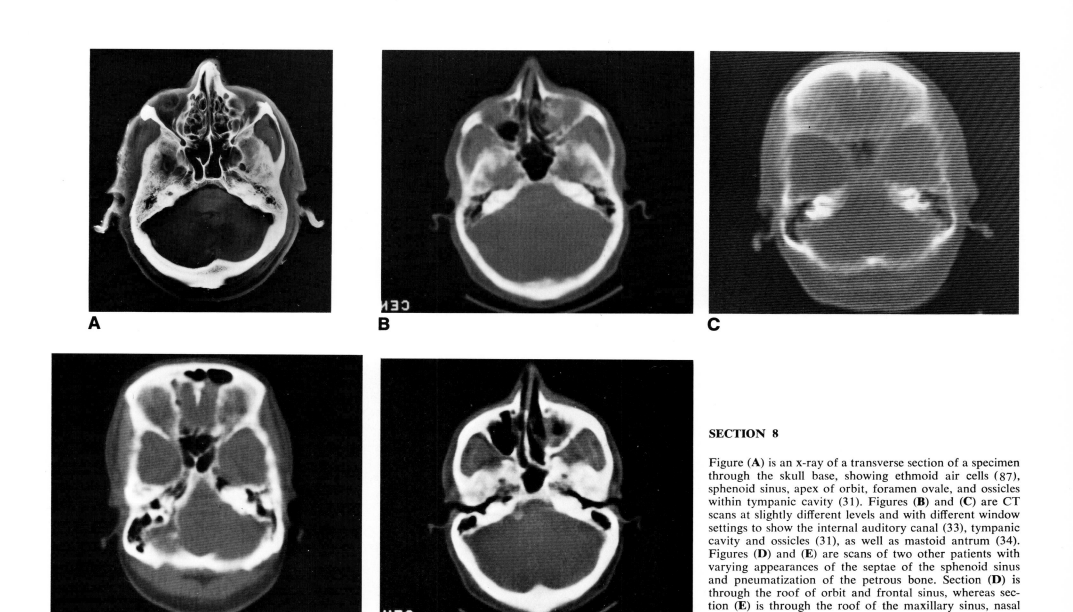

A

B

C

D

E

SECTION 8

Figure (**A**) is an x-ray of a transverse section of a specimen through the skull base, showing ethmoid air cells (87), sphenoid sinus, apex of orbit, foramen ovale, and ossicles within tympanic cavity (31). Figures (**B**) and (**C**) are CT scans at slightly different levels and with different window settings to show the internal auditory canal (33), tympanic cavity and ossicles (31), as well as mastoid antrum (34). Figures (**D**) and (**E**) are scans of two other patients with varying appearances of the septae of the sphenoid sinus and pneumatization of the petrous bone. Section (**D**) is through the roof of orbit and frontal sinus, whereas section (**E**) is through the roof of the maxillary sinus, nasal cavity, and sphenoid sinus.

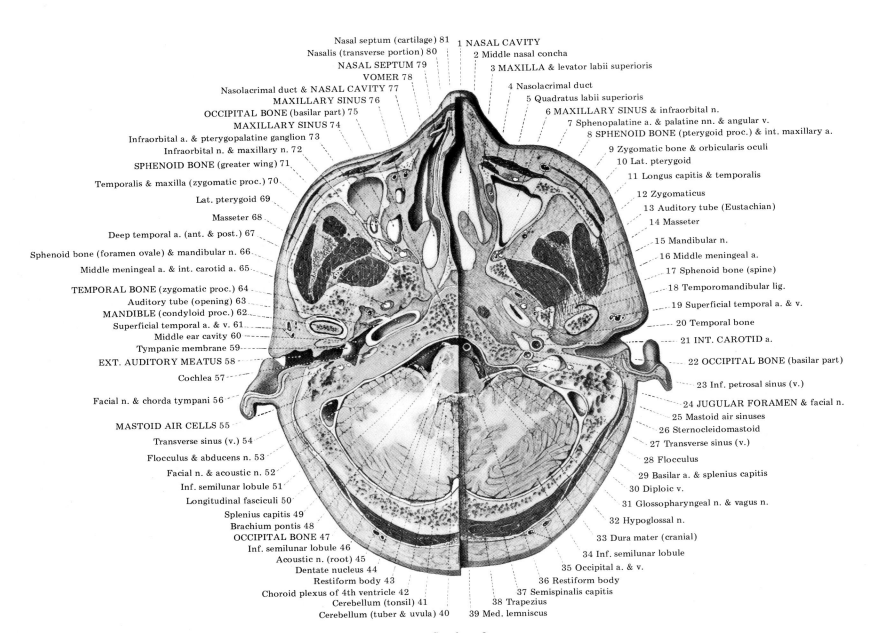

Nasal septum (cartilage) 81
Nasalis (transverse portion) 80
NASAL SEPTUM 79
VOMER 78
Nasolacrimal duct & NASAL CAVITY 77
MAXILLARY SINUS 76
OCCIPITAL BONE (basilar part) 75
MAXILLARY SINUS 74
Infraorbital a. & pterygopalatine ganglion 73
Infraorbital n. & maxillary n. 72
SPHENOID BONE (greater wing) 71
Temporalis & maxilla (zygomatic proc.) 70
Lat. pterygoid 69
Masseter 68
Deep temporal a. (ant. & post.) 67
Sphenoid bone (foramen ovale) & mandibular n. 66
Middle meningeal a. & int. carotid a. 65
TEMPORAL BONE (zygomatic proc.) 64
Auditory tube (opening) 63
MANDIBLE (condyloid proc.) 62
Superficial temporal a. & v. 61
Middle ear cavity 60
Tympanic membrane 59
EXT. AUDITORY MEATUS 58
Cochlea 57
Facial n. & chorda tympani 56
MASTOID AIR CELLS 55
Transverse sinus (v.) 54
Flocculus & abducens n. 53
Facial n. & acoustic n. 52
Inf. semilunar lobule 51
Longitudinal fasciculi 50
Splenius capitis 49
Brachium pontis 48
OCCIPITAL BONE 47
Inf. semilunar lobule 46
Acoustic n. (root) 45
Dentate nucleus 44
Restiform body 43
Choroid plexus of 4th ventricle 42
Cerebellum (tonsil) 41
Cerebellum (tuber & uvula) 40

1 NASAL CAVITY
2 Middle nasal concha
3 MAXILLA & levator labii superioris
4 Nasolacrimal duct
5 Quadratus labii superioris
6 MAXILLARY SINUS & infraorbital n.
7 Sphenopalatine a. & palatine nn. & angular v.
8 SPHENOID BONE (pterygoid proc.) & int. maxillary a.
9 Zygomatic bone & orbicularis oculi
10 Lat. pterygoid
11 Longus capitis & temporalis
12 Zygomaticus
13 Auditory tube (Eustachian)
14 Masseter
15 Mandibular n.
16 Middle meningeal a.
17 Sphenoid bone (spine)
18 Temporomandibular lig.
19 Superficial temporal a. & v.
20 Temporal bone
21 INT. CAROTID a.
22 OCCIPITAL BONE (basilar part)
23 Inf. petrosal sinus (v.)
24 JUGULAR FORAMEN & facial n.
25 Mastoid air sinuses
26 Sternocleidomastoid
27 Transverse sinus (v.)
28 Flocculus
29 Basilar a. & splenius capitis
30 Diploic v.
31 Glossopharyngeal n. & vagus n.
32 Hypoglossal n.
33 Dura mater (cranial)
34 Inf. semilunar lobule
35 Occipital a. & v.
36 Restiform body
37 Semispinalis capitis
38 Trapezius
39 Med. lemniscus

Section 9

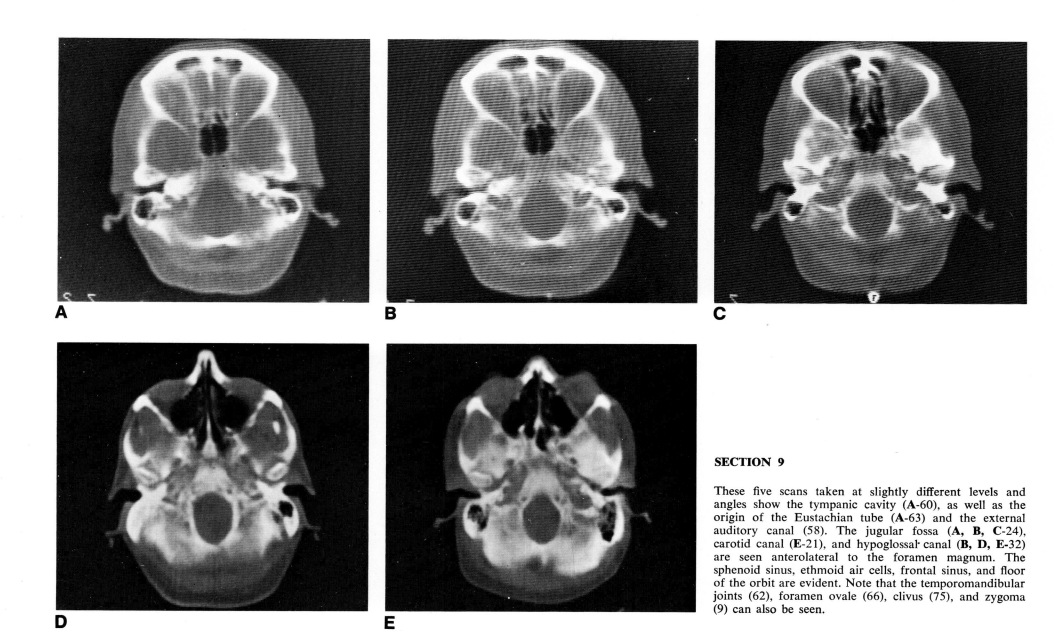

A **B** **C**

D **E**

SECTION 9

These five scans taken at slightly different levels and angles show the tympanic cavity (**A**-60), as well as the origin of the Eustachian tube (**A**-63) and the external auditory canal (58). The jugular fossa (**A, B, C**-24), carotid canal (**E**-21), and hypoglossal canal (**B, D, E**-32) are seen anterolateral to the foramen magnum. The sphenoid sinus, ethmoid air cells, frontal sinus, and floor of the orbit are evident. Note that the temporomandibular joints (62), foramen ovale (66), clivus (75), and zygoma (9) can also be seen.

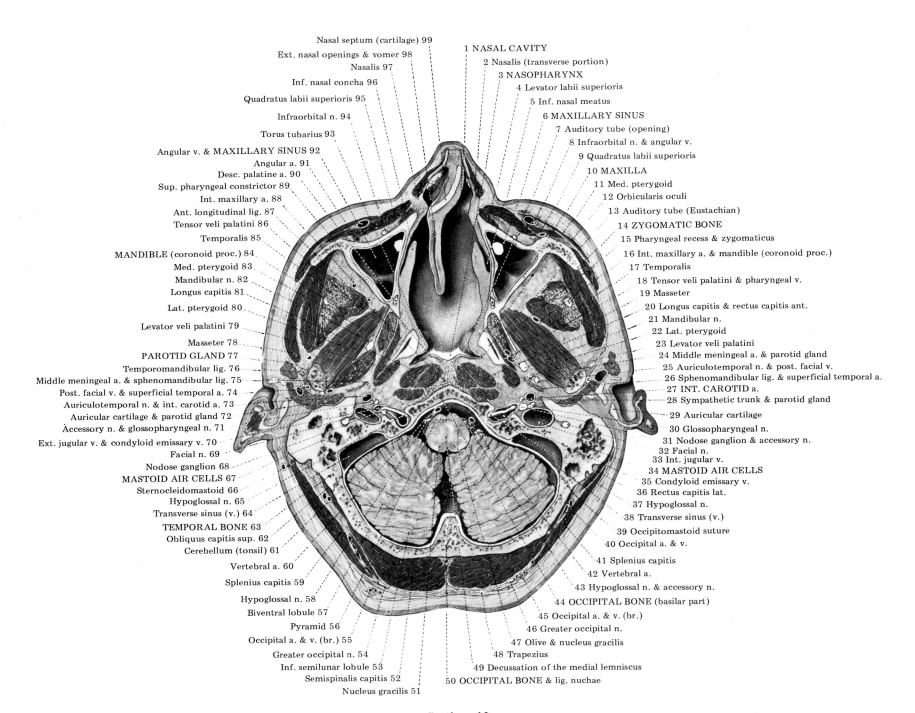

Nasal septum (cartilage) 99
Ext. nasal openings & vomer 98
Nasalis 97
Inf. nasal concha 96
Quadratus labii superioris 95
Infraorbital n. 94
Torus tubarius 93
Angular v. & MAXILLARY SINUS 92
Angular a. 91
Desc. palatine a. 90
Sup. pharyngeal constrictor 89
Int. maxillary a. 88
Ant. longitudinal lig. 87
Tensor veli palatini 86
Temporalis 85
MANDIBLE (coronoid proc.) 84
Med. pterygoid 83
Mandibular n. 82
Longus capitis 81
Lat. pterygoid 80
Levator veli palatini 79
Masseter 78
PAROTID GLAND 77
Temporomandibular lig. 76
Middle meningeal a. & sphenomandibular lig. 75
Post. facial v. & superficial temporal a. 74
Auriculotemporal n. & int. carotid a. 73
Auricular cartilage & parotid gland 72
Accessory n. & glossopharyngeal n. 71
Ext. jugular v. & condyloid emissary v. 70
Facial n. 69
Nodose ganglion 68
MASTOID AIR CELLS 67
Sternocleidomastoid 66
Hypoglossal n. 65
Transverse sinus (v.) 64
TEMPORAL BONE 63
Obliquus capitis sup. 62
Cerebellum (tonsil) 61
Vertebral a. 60
Splenius capitis 59
Hypoglossal n. 58
Biventral lobule 57
Pyramid 56
Occipital a. & v. (br.) 55
Greater occipital n. 54
Inf. semilunar lobule 53
Semispinalis capitis 52
Nucleus gracilis 51

1 NASAL CAVITY
2 Nasalis (transverse portion)
3 NASOPHARYNX
4 Levator labii superioris
5 Inf. nasal meatus
6 MAXILLARY SINUS
7 Auditory tube (opening)
8 Infraorbital n. & angular v.
9 Quadratus labii superioris
10 MAXILLA
11 Med. pterygoid
12 Orbicularis oculi
13 Auditory tube (Eustachian)
14 ZYGOMATIC BONE
15 Pharyngeal recess & zygomaticus
16 Int. maxillary a. & mandible (coronoid proc.)
17 Temporalis
18 Tensor veli palatini & pharyngeal v.
19 Masseter
20 Longus capitis & rectus capitis ant.
21 Mandibular n.
22 Lat. pterygoid
23 Levator veli palatini
24 Middle meningeal a. & parotid gland
25 Auriculotemporal n. & post. facial v.
26 Sphenomandibular lig. & superficial temporal a.
27 INT. CAROTID a.
28 Sympathetic trunk & parotid gland
29 Auricular cartilage
30 Glossopharyngeal n.
31 Nodose ganglion & accessory n.
32 Facial n.
33 Int. jugular v.
34 MASTOID AIR CELLS
35 Condyloid emissary v.
36 Rectus capitis lat.
37 Hypoglossal n.
38 Transverse sinus (v.)
39 Occipitomastoid suture
40 Occipital a. & v.
41 Splenius capitis
42 Vertebral a.
43 Hypoglossal n. & accessory n.
44 OCCIPITAL BONE (basilar part)
45 Occipital a. & v. (br.)
46 Greater occipital n.
47 Olive & nucleus gracilis
48 Trapezius
49 Decussation of the medial lemniscus
50 OCCIPITAL BONE & lig. nuchae

Section 10

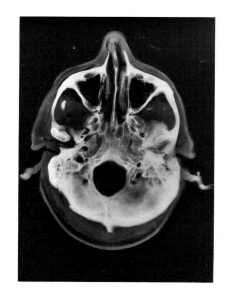

A

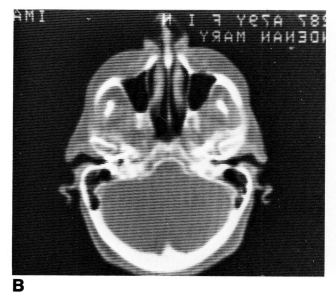

B

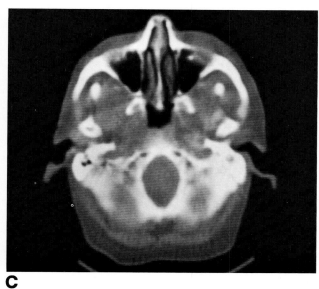

C

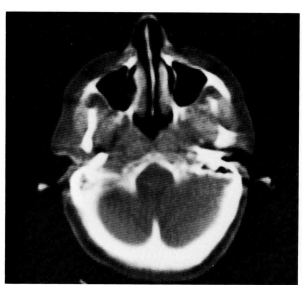

D

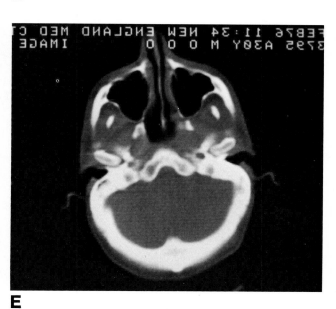

E

SECTION 10

The maxillary sinuses (6) and nasal cavity (1) are clearly visualized on specimen (**A**) and CT scans (**B** through **E**). Soft-tissue detail of CT scanning permits visualization of the lateral pterygoid muscle (80), masseter muscles (19), and nasopharynx (3). Bone detail is also sharply defined with pneumatized mastoid air cells (**B-67**), transverse sinus (**B-64**), mandibular condyle, coronoid process (84), zygoma (14), and pterygoid plates. The jugular fossa (33) and carotid canal (27) are evident.

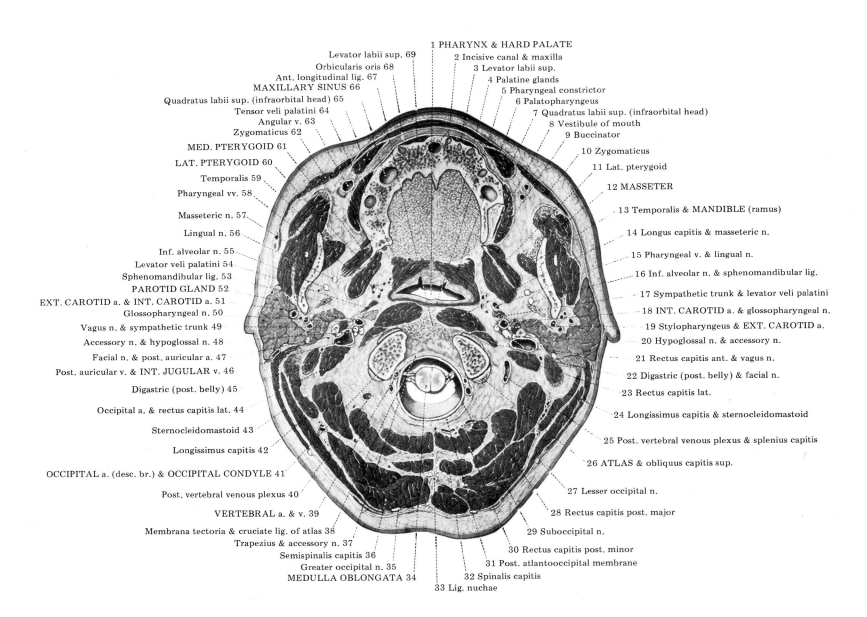

1 PHARYNX & HARD PALATE
2 Incisive canal & maxilla
3 Levator labii sup.
4 Palatine glands
5 Pharyngeal constrictor
6 Palatopharyngeus
7 Quadratus labii sup. (infraorbital head)
8 Vestibule of mouth
9 Buccinator
10 Zygomaticus
11 Lat. pterygoid
12 MASSETER
13 Temporalis & MANDIBLE (ramus)
14 Longus capitis & masseteric n.
15 Pharyngeal v. & lingual n.
16 Inf. alveolar n. & sphenomandibular lig.
17 Sympathetic trunk & levator veli palatini
18 INT. CAROTID a. & glossopharyngeal n.
19 Stylopharyngeus & EXT. CAROTID a.
20 Hypoglossal n. & accessory n.
21 Rectus capitis ant. & vagus n.
22 Digastric (post. belly) & facial n.
23 Rectus capitis lat.
24 Longissimus capitis & sternocleidomastoid
25 Post. vertebral venous plexus & splenius capitis
26 ATLAS & obliquus capitis sup.
27 Lesser occipital n.
28 Rectus capitis post. major
29 Suboccipital n.
30 Rectus capitis post. minor
31 Post. atlantooccipital membrane
32 Spinalis capitis
33 Lig. nuchae
MEDULLA OBLONGATA 34
Greater occipital n. 35
Semispinalis capitis 36
Trapezius & accessory n. 37
Membrana tectoria & cruciate lig. of atlas 38
VERTEBRAL a. & v. 39
Post. vertebral venous plexus 40
OCCIPITAL a. (desc. br.) & OCCIPITAL CONDYLE 41
Longissimus capitis 42
Sternocleidomastoid 43
Occipital a. & rectus capitis lat. 44
Digastric (post. belly) 45
Post. auricular v. & INT. JUGULAR v. 46
Facial n. & post. auricular a. 47
Accessory n. & hypoglossal n. 48
Vagus n. & sympathetic trunk 49
Glossopharyngeal n. 50
EXT. CAROTID a. & INT. CAROTID a. 51
PAROTID GLAND 52
Sphenomandibular lig. 53
Levator veli palatini 54
Inf. alveolar n. 55
Lingual n. 56
Masseteric n. 57
Pharyngeal vv. 58
Temporalis 59
LAT. PTERYGOID 60
MED. PTERYGOID 61
Zygomaticus 62
Angular v. 63
Tensor veli palatini 64
Quadratus labii sup. (infraorbital head) 65
MAXILLARY SINUS 66
Ant. longitudinal lig. 67
Orbicularis oris 68
Levator labii sup. 69

Section 11

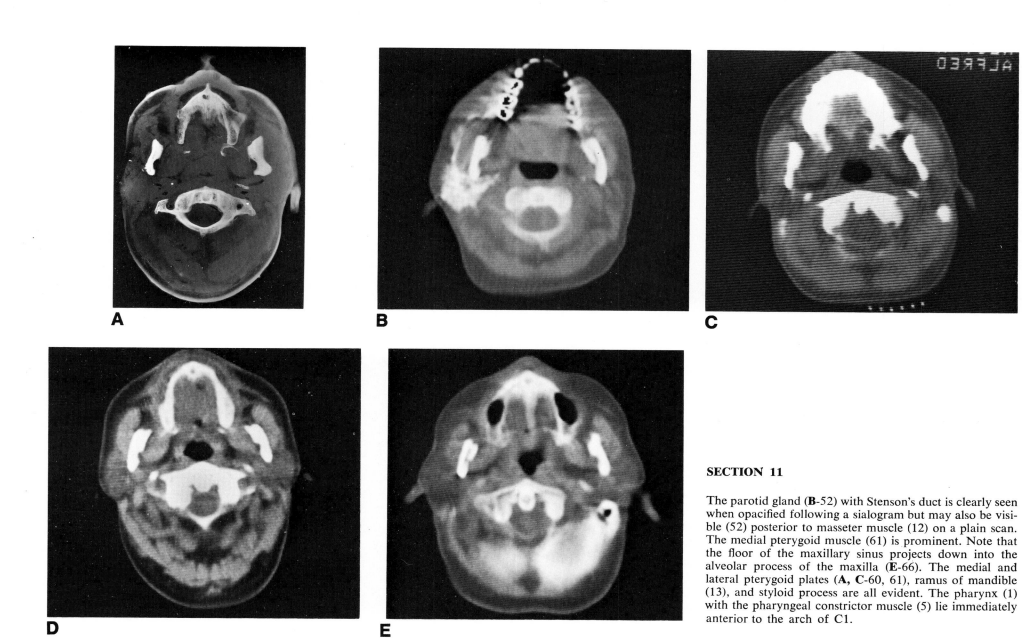

A **B** **C**

D **E**

SECTION 11

The parotid gland (**B**-52) with Stenson's duct is clearly seen
when opacified following a sialogram but may also be visible (52) posterior to masseter muscle (12) on a plain scan.
The medial pterygoid muscle (61) is prominent. Note that
the floor of the maxillary sinus projects down into the
alveolar process of the maxilla (**E**-66). The medial and
lateral pterygoid plates (**A, C**-60, 61), ramus of mandible
(13), and styloid process are all evident. The pharynx (1)
with the pharyngeal constrictor muscle (5) lie immediately
anterior to the arch of C1.

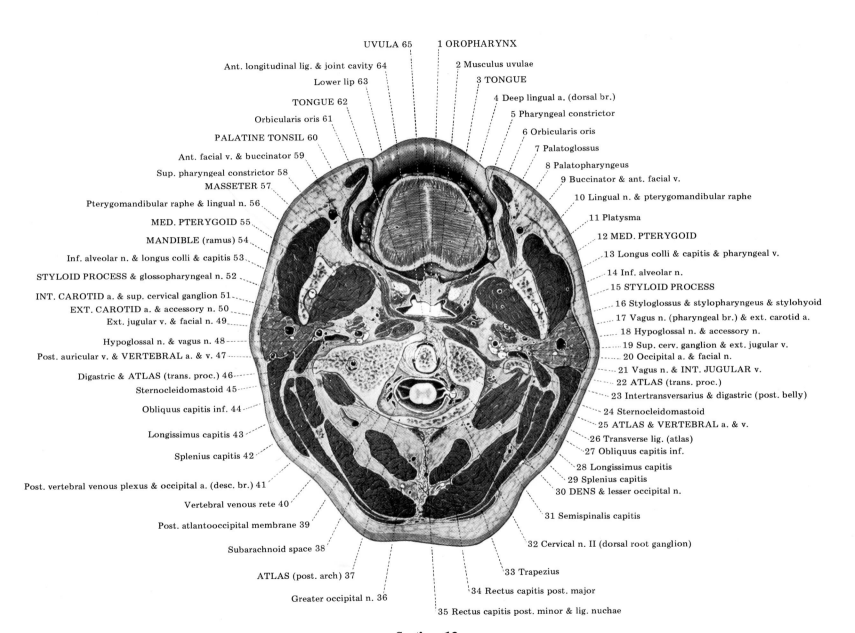

UVULA 65   1 OROPHARYNX

Ant. longitudinal lig. & joint cavity 64

2 Musculus uvulae

Lower lip 63

3 TONGUE

TONGUE 62

4 Deep lingual a. (dorsal br.)

Orbicularis oris 61

5 Pharyngeal constrictor

PALATINE TONSIL 60

6 Orbicularis oris

Ant. facial v. & buccinator 59

7 Palatoglossus

8 Palatopharyngeus

Sup. pharyngeal constrictor 58

9 Buccinator & ant. facial v.

MASSETER 57

10 Lingual n. & pterygomandibular raphe

Pterygomandibular raphe & lingual n. 56

11 Platysma

MED. PTERYGOID 55

12 MED. PTERYGOID

MANDIBLE (ramus) 54

13 Longus colli & capitis & pharyngeal v.

Inf. alveolar n. & longus colli & capitis 53

14 Inf. alveolar n.

STYLOID PROCESS & glossopharyngeal n. 52

15 STYLOID PROCESS

INT. CAROTID a. & sup. cervical ganglion 51

16 Styloglossus & stylopharyngeus & stylohyoid

EXT. CAROTID a. & accessory n. 50

17 Vagus n. (pharyngeal br.) & ext. carotid a.

Ext. jugular v. & facial n. 49

18 Hypoglossal n. & accessory n.

Hypoglossal n. & vagus n. 48

19 Sup. cerv. ganglion & ext. jugular v.

Post. auricular v. & VERTEBRAL a. & v. 47

20 Occipital a. & facial n.

21 Vagus n. & INT. JUGULAR v.

Digastric & ATLAS (trans. proc.) 46

22 ATLAS (trans. proc.)

23 Intertransversarius & digastric (post. belly)

Sternocleidomastoid 45

24 Sternocleidomastoid

Obliquus capitis inf. 44

25 ATLAS & VERTEBRAL a. & v.

26 Transverse lig. (atlas)

27 Obliquus capitis inf.

Longissimus capitis 43

28 Longissimus capitis

Splenius capitis 42

29 Splenius capitis

30 DENS & lesser occipital n.

Post. vertebral venous plexus & occipital a. (desc. br.) 41

31 Semispinalis capitis

Vertebral venous rete 40

32 Cervical n. II (dorsal root ganglion)

Post. atlantooccipital membrane 39

Subarachnoid space 38

33 Trapezius

ATLAS (post. arch) 37

34 Rectus capitis post. major

Greater occipital n. 36

35 Rectus capitis post. minor & lig. nuchae

Section 12

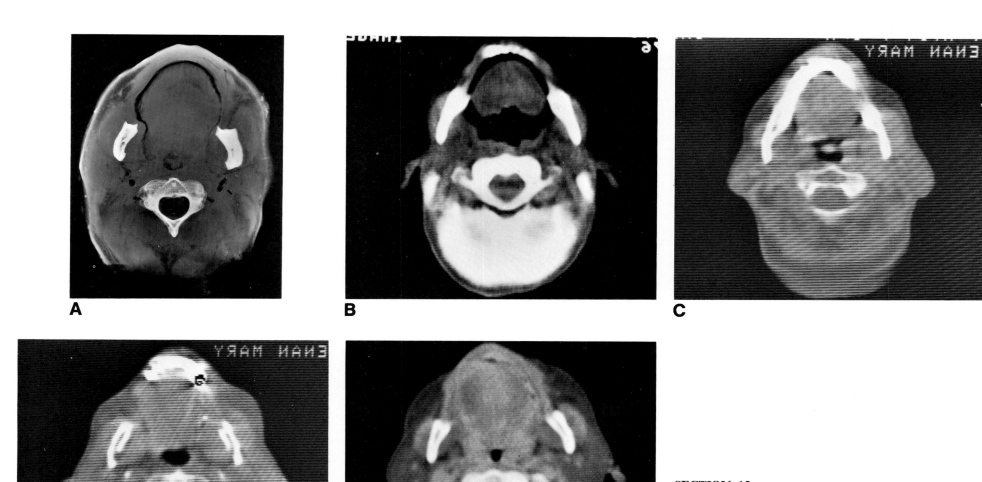

A

B

C

D

E

SECTION 12

The oropharynx (1), palatine tonsils (C-60), and uvula (A, C-65) are seen at the same level as the tongue (3). The styloid process (D-15) is medial to the medial pterygoid muscle (12) and ramus of the mandible (54). The masseter muscle (57) is prominent. The jugular veins and carotid arteries (21, 50, 51) lie deep to the parotid gland and appear slightly dense on the CT scans (C) and (E) but are filled with air in the specimen (A).

Section 12

TONSIL

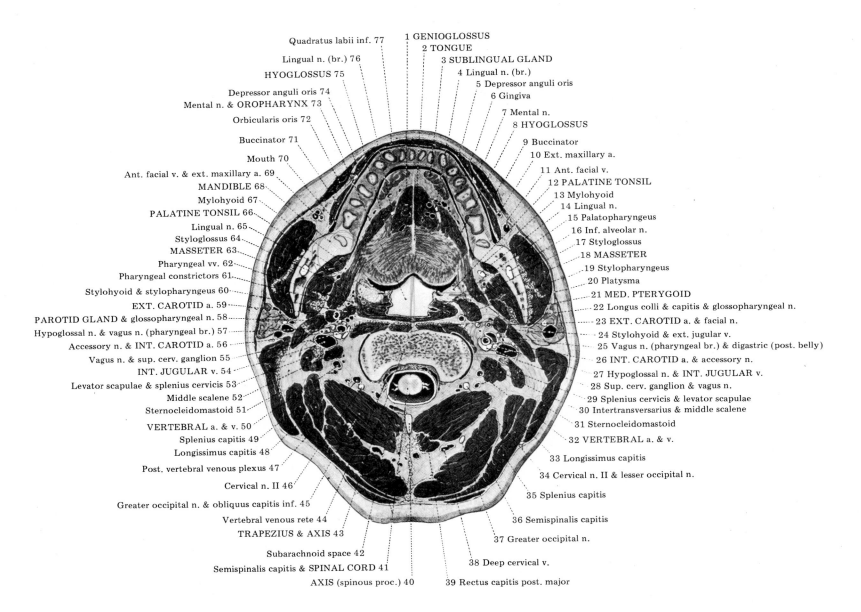

Quadratus labii inf. 77
1 GENIOGLOSSUS
2 TONGUE
Lingual n. (br.) 76
3 SUBLINGUAL GLAND
HYOGLOSSUS 75
4 Lingual n. (br.)
5 Depressor anguli oris
Depressor anguli oris 74
6 Gingiva
Mental n. & OROPHARYNX 73
Orbicularis oris 72
7 Mental n.
8 HYOGLOSSUS
Buccinator 71
9 Buccinator
Mouth 70
10 Ext. maxillary a.
Ant. facial v. & ext. maxillary a. 69
11 Ant. facial v.
MANDIBLE 68
12 PALATINE TONSIL
Mylohyoid 67
13 Mylohyoid
PALATINE TONSIL 66
14 Lingual n.
Lingual n. 65
15 Palatopharyngeus
Styloglossus 64
16 Inf. alveolar n.
MASSETER 63
17 Styloglossus
Pharyngeal vv. 62
18 MASSETER
Pharyngeal constrictors 61
19 Stylopharyngeus
Stylohyoid & stylopharyngeus 60
20 Platysma
EXT. CAROTID a. 59
21 MED. PTERYGOID
PAROTID GLAND & glossopharyngeal n. 58
22 Longus colli & capitis & glossopharyngeal n.
Hypoglossal n. & vagus n. (pharyngeal br.) 57
23 EXT. CAROTID a. & facial n.
Accessory n. & INT. CAROTID a. 56
24 Stylohyoid & ext. jugular v.
Vagus n. & sup. cerv. ganglion 55
25 Vagus n. (pharyngeal br.) & digastric (post. belly)
INT. JUGULAR v. 54
26 INT. CAROTID a. & accessory n.
Levator scapulae & splenius cervicis 53
27 Hypoglossal n. & INT. JUGULAR v.
Middle scalene 52
28 Sup. cerv. ganglion & vagus n.
Sternocleidomastoid 51
29 Splenius cervicis & levator scapulae
30 Intertransversarius & middle scalene
VERTEBRAL a. & v. 50
31 Sternocleidomastoid
Splenius capitis 49
32 VERTEBRAL a. & v.
Longissimus capitis 48
33 Longissimus capitis
Post. vertebral venous plexus 47
34 Cervical n. II & lesser occipital n.
Cervical n. II 46
35 Splenius capitis
Greater occipital n. & obliquus capitis inf. 45
36 Semispinalis capitis
Vertebral venous rete 44
37 Greater occipital n.
TRAPEZIUS & AXIS 43
Subarachnoid space 42
38 Deep cervical v.
Semispinalis capitis & SPINAL CORD 41
39 Rectus capitis post. major
AXIS (spinous proc.) 40

Section 13

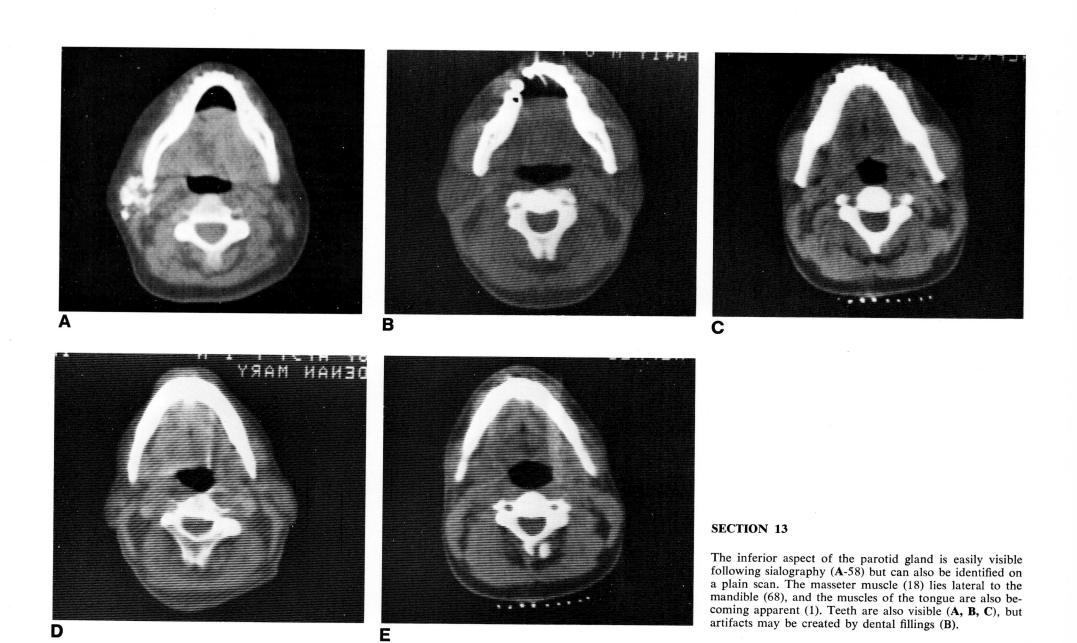

A

B

C

D

E

SECTION 13

The inferior aspect of the parotid gland is easily visible following sialography (A-58) but can also be identified on a plain scan. The masseter muscle (18) lies lateral to the mandible (68), and the muscles of the tongue are also becoming apparent (1). Teeth are also visible (**A, B, C**), but artifacts may be created by dental fillings (**B**).

Section 13

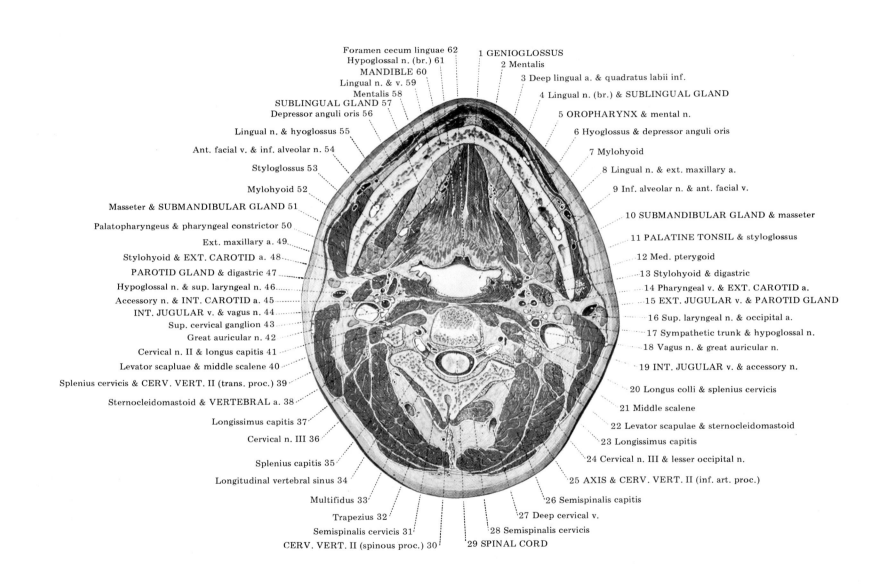

Foramen cecum linguae 62
Hypoglossal n. (br.) 61
MANDIBLE 60
Lingual n. & v. 59
Mentalis 58
SUBLINGUAL GLAND 57
Depressor anguli oris 56
Lingual n. & hyoglossus 55
Ant. facial v. & inf. alveolar n. 54
Styloglossus 53
Mylohyoid 52
Masseter & SUBMANDIBULAR GLAND 51
Palatopharyngeus & pharyngeal constrictor 50
Ext. maxillary a. 49
Stylohyoid & EXT. CAROTID a. 48
PAROTID GLAND & digastric 47
Hypoglossal n. & sup. laryngeal n. 46
Accessory n. & INT. CAROTID a. 45
INT. JUGULAR v. & vagus n. 44
Sup. cervical ganglion 43
Great auricular n. 42
Cervical n. II & longus capitis 41
Levator scapluae & middle scalene 40
Splenius cervicis & CERV. VERT. II (trans. proc.) 39
Sternocleidomastoid & VERTEBRAL a. 38
Longissimus capitis 37
Cervical n. III 36
Splenius capitis 35
Longitudinal vertebral sinus 34
Multifidus 33
Trapezius 32
Semispinalis cervicis 31
CERV. VERT. II (spinous proc.) 30

1 GENIOGLOSSUS
2 Mentalis
3 Deep lingual a. & quadratus labii inf.
4 Lingual n. (br.) & SUBLINGUAL GLAND
5 OROPHARYNX & mental n.
6 Hyoglossus & depressor anguli oris
7 Mylohyoid
8 Lingual n. & ext. maxillary a.
9 Inf. alveolar n. & ant. facial v.
10 SUBMANDIBULAR GLAND & masseter
11 PALATINE TONSIL & styloglossus
12 Med. pterygoid
13 Stylohyoid & digastric
14 Pharyngeal v. & EXT. CAROTID a.
15 EXT. JUGULAR v. & PAROTID GLAND
16 Sup. laryngeal n. & occipital a.
17 Sympathetic trunk & hypoglossal n.
18 Vagus n. & great auricular n.
19 INT. JUGULAR v. & accessory n.
20 Longus colli & splenius cervicis
21 Middle scalene
22 Levator scapulae & sternocleidomastoid
23 Longissimus capitis
24 Cervical n. III & lesser occipital n.
25 AXIS & CERV. VERT. II (inf. art. proc.)
26 Semispinalis capitis
27 Deep cervical v.
28 Semispinalis cervicis
29 SPINAL CORD

Section 14

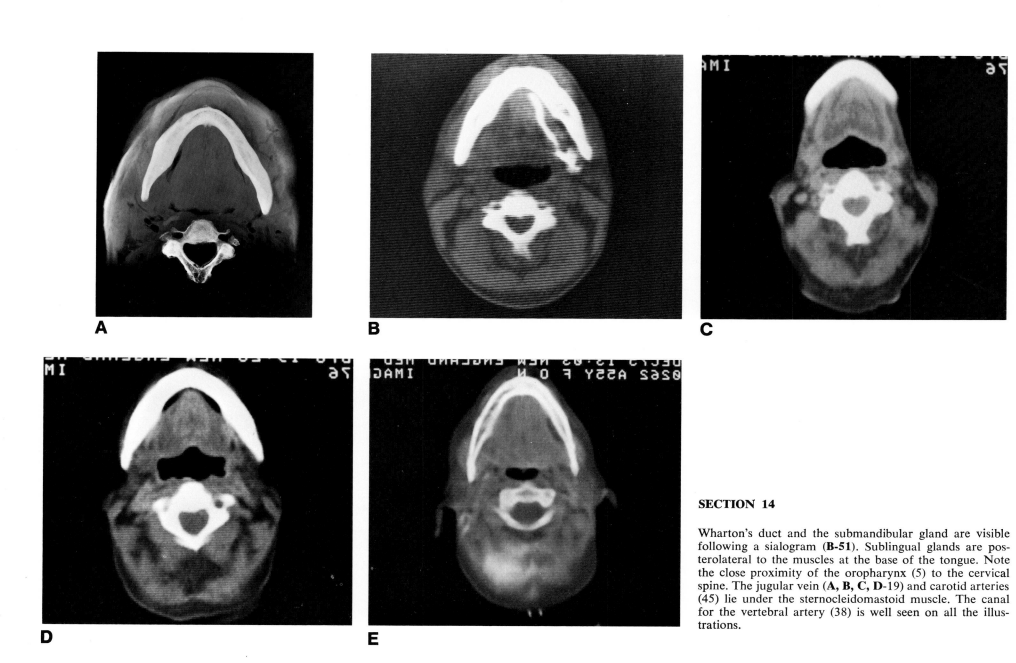

A

B

C

D

E

SECTION 14

Wharton's duct and the submandibular gland are visible following a sialogram (**B**-51). Sublingual glands are posterolateral to the muscles at the base of the tongue. Note the close proximity of the oropharynx (5) to the cervical spine. The jugular vein (**A, B, C, D**-19) and carotid arteries (45) lie under the sternocleidomastoid muscle. The canal for the vertebral artery (38) is well seen on all the illustrations.

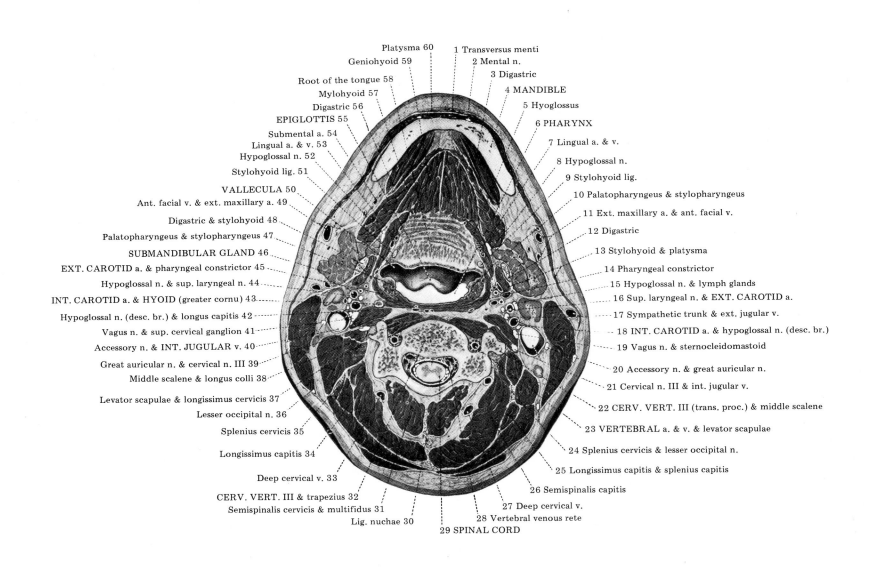

Platysma 60

Geniohyoid 59

Root of the tongue 58

Mylohyoid 57

Digastric 56

EPIGLOTTIS 55

Submental a. 54

Lingual a. & v. 53

Hypoglossal n. 52

Stylohyoid lig. 51

VALLECULA 50

Ant. facial v. & ext. maxillary a. 49

Digastric & stylohyoid 48

Palatopharyngeus & stylopharyngeus 47

SUBMANDIBULAR GLAND 46

EXT. CAROTID a. & pharyngeal constrictor 45

Hypoglossal n. & sup. laryngeal n. 44

INT. CAROTID a. & HYOID (greater cornu) 43

Hypoglossal n. (desc. br.) & longus capitis 42

Vagus n. & sup. cervical ganglion 41

Accessory n. & INT. JUGULAR v. 40

Great auricular n. & cervical n. III 39

Middle scalene & longus colli 38

Levator scapulae & longissimus cervicis 37

Lesser occipital n. 36

Splenius cervicis 35

Longissimus capitis 34

Deep cervical v. 33

CERV. VERT. III & trapezius 32

Semispinalis cervicis & multifidus 31

Lig. nuchae 30

29 SPINAL CORD

1 Transversus menti

2 Mental n.

3 Digastric

4 MANDIBLE

5 Hyoglossus

6 PHARYNX

7 Lingual a. & v.

8 Hypoglossal n.

9 Stylohyoid lig.

10 Palatopharyngeus & stylopharyngeus

11 Ext. maxillary a. & ant. facial v.

12 Digastric

13 Stylohyoid & platysma

14 Pharyngeal constrictor

15 Hypoglossal n. & lymph glands

16 Sup. laryngeal n. & EXT. CAROTID a.

17 Sympathetic trunk & ext. jugular v.

18 INT. CAROTID a. & hypoglossal n. (desc. br.)

19 Vagus n. & sternocleidomastoid

20 Accessory n. & great auricular n.

21 Cervical n. III & int. jugular v.

22 CERV. VERT. III (trans. proc.) & middle scalene

23 VERTEBRAL a. & v. & levator scapulae

24 Splenius cervicis & lesser occipital n.

25 Longissimus capitis & splenius capitis

26 Semispinalis capitis

27 Deep cervical v.

28 Vertebral venous rete

Section 15

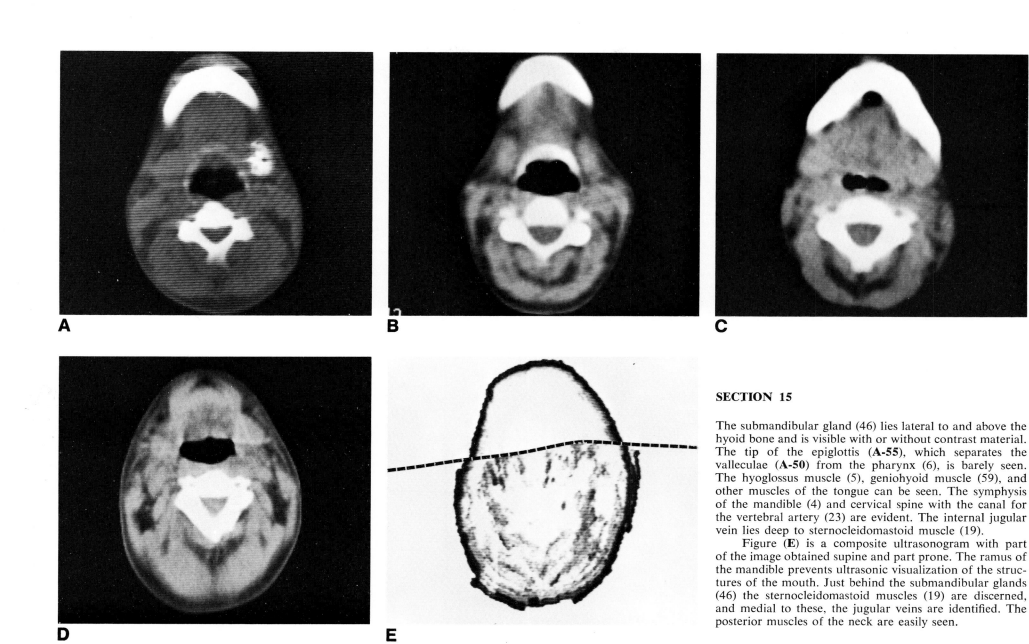

A

B

C

D

E

SECTION 15

The submandibular gland (46) lies lateral to and above the hyoid bone and is visible with or without contrast material. The tip of the epiglottis (A-55), which separates the valleculae (A-50) from the pharynx (6), is barely seen. The hyoglossus muscle (5), geniohyoid muscle (59), and other muscles of the tongue can be seen. The symphysis of the mandible (4) and cervical spine with the canal for the vertebral artery (23) are evident. The internal jugular vein lies deep to sternocleidomastoid muscle (19).

Figure (E) is a composite ultrasonogram with part of the image obtained supine and part prone. The ramus of the mandible prevents ultrasonic visualization of the structures of the mouth. Just behind the submandibular glands (46) the sternocleidomastoid muscles (19) are discerned, and medial to these, the jugular veins are identified. The posterior muscles of the neck are easily seen.

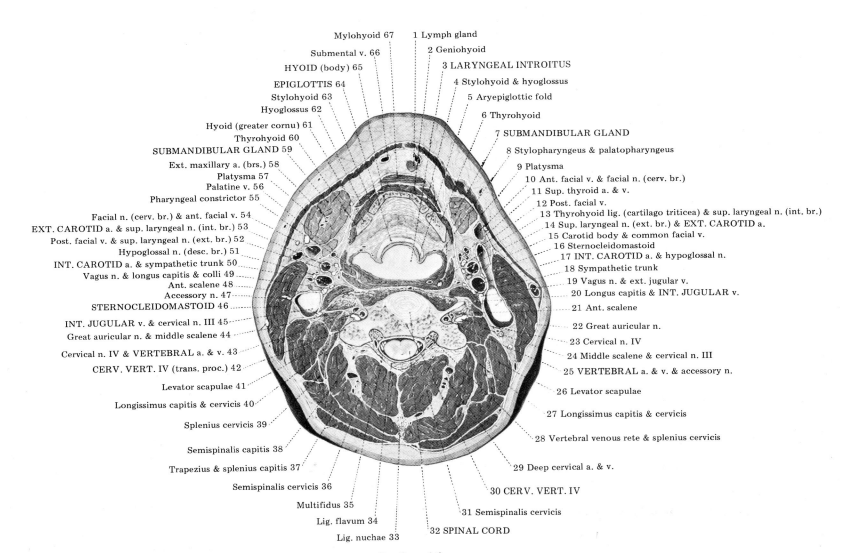

Mylohyoid 67
Submental v. 66
HYOID (body) 65
EPIGLOTTIS 64
Stylohyoid 63
Hyoglossus 62
Hyoid (greater cornu) 61
Thyrohyoid 60
SUBMANDIBULAR GLAND 59
Ext. maxillary a. (brs.) 58
Platysma 57
Palatine v. 56
Pharyngeal constrictor 55
Facial n. (cerv. br.) & ant. facial v. 54
EXT. CAROTID a. & sup. laryngeal n. (int. br.) 53
Post. facial v. & sup. laryngeal n. (ext. br.) 52
Hypoglossal n. (desc. br.) 51
INT. CAROTID a. & sympathetic trunk 50
Vagus n. & longus capitis & colli 49
Ant. scalene 48
Accessory n. 47
STERNOCLEIDOMASTOID 46
INT. JUGULAR v. & cervical n. III 45
Great auricular n. & middle scalene 44
Cervical n. IV & VERTEBRAL a. & v. 43
CERV. VERT. IV (trans. proc.) 42
Levator scapulae 41
Longissimus capitis & cervicis 40
Splenius cervicis 39
Semispinalis capitis 38
Trapezius & splenius capitis 37
Semispinalis cervicis 36
Multifidus 35
Lig. flavum 34
Lig. nuchae 33

1 Lymph gland
2 Geniohyoid
3 LARYNGEAL INTROITUS
4 Stylohyoid & hyoglossus
5 Aryepiglottic fold
6 Thyrohyoid
7 SUBMANDIBULAR GLAND
8 Stylopharyngeus & palatopharyngeus
9 Platysma
10 Ant. facial v. & facial n. (cerv. br.)
11 Sup. thyroid a. & v.
12 Post. facial v.
13 Thyrohyoid lig. (cartilago triticea) & sup. laryngeal n. (int. br.)
14 Sup. laryngeal n. (ext. br.) & EXT. CAROTID a.
15 Carotid body & common facial v.
16 Sternocleidomastoid
17 INT. CAROTID a. & hypoglossal n.
18 Sympathetic trunk
19 Vagus n. & ext. jugular v.
20 Longus capitis & INT. JUGULAR v.
21 Ant. scalene
22 Great auricular n.
23 Cervical n. IV
24 Middle scalene & cervical n. III
25 VERTEBRAL a. & v. & accessory n.
26 Levator scapulae
27 Longissimus capitis & cervicis
28 Vertebral venous rete & splenius cervicis
29 Deep cervical a. & v.
30 CERV. VERT. IV
31 Semispinalis cervicis
32 SPINAL CORD

Section 16

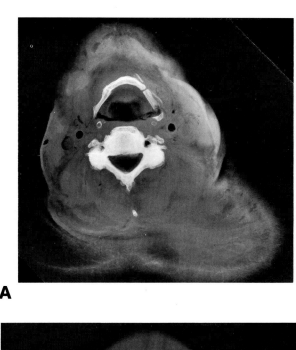

A

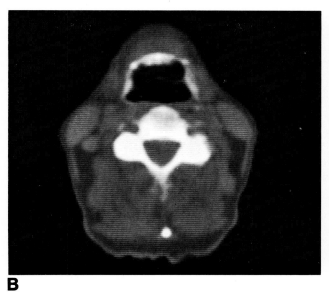

B

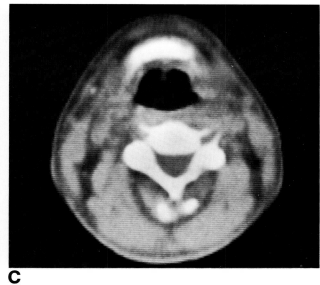

C

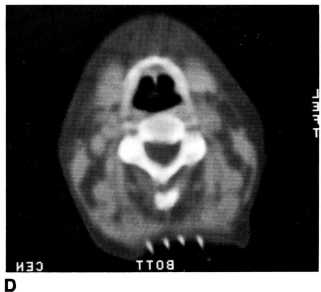

D

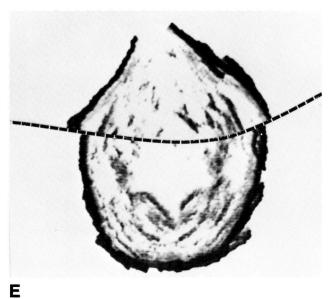

E

SECTION 16

The specimen and scans taken at the level of the hyoid bone (65) again show the submandibular gland (**D**-59), valleculae, epiglottis (64), and hypopharynx (3). The internal jugular vein (45) and carotid artery (17), which are filled with air on the specimen (**A**) and with blood on CT scans, are located under the sternocleidomastoid muscle (46). Note the canal for the vertebral artery and vein (25).

Figure (**E**) is a composite anterior and posterior ultrasonogram. Very little definite structure is seen in the upper neck. Laterally, the sternomastoid muscles (46) are well defined, and the large internal jugular veins (45) are seen, with the internal carotid artery (17) also identifiable. The posterior muscles of the neck stand out clearly. There are no echoes from inside the spine.

CORNICULATE CARTILAGE 58
Platysma & THYROID CARTILAGE (left lamina) 57
HYPOPHARYNX 56
Thyrohyoid 55
Sup. laryngeal n. (int. br.) 54
Pharyngeal constrictor 53
Common facial v. & sup. thyroid a. 52
Longus colli & capitis 51
COMMON CAROTID a. & sympathetic trunk 50
Hypoglossal n. (desc. br.) 49
Vagus n. & ant. scalene 48
INT. JUGULAR v. & VERTEBRAL a. & v. 47
Cervical n. IV 46
Cervical n. III 45
Great auricular n. 44
Accessory n. & levator scapulae 43
Longissimus cervicis 42
CERV. VERT. IV (inf. art. proc.) 41
Longissimus capitis & cervical n. V 40
Splenius cervicis 39
Deep cervical a. & v. 38
Trapezius 37
Splenius capitis 36
Semispinalis capitis 35
Multifidus 34
Semispinalis cervicis 33
CERV. VERT. IV (spinous proc.) 32
Lig. nuchae 31

1 Ant. jugular v.
2 EPIGLOTTIS
3 LARYNX (vestibule)
4 Sternohyoid & omohyoid
5 Sup. laryngeal n. (int. br.)
6 Platysma
7 Communicating v.
8 Inf. pharyngeal constrictor
9 THYROID CARTILAGE (sup. horn)
10 Sympathetic trunk & COMMON CAROTID a.
11 Hypoglossal n. (desc. br.)
12 Longus colli & capitis
13 Ant. scalene & vagus n.
14 STERNOCLEIDOMASTOID & ext. jugular v.
15 CERV. VERT. IV (trans. proc.)
16 Middle scalene & cervical n. IV
17 CERV. VERT. V (sup. art. proc.) & cervical n. III
18 Cervical n. V & accessory n.
19 Levator scapulae
20 Post. longitudinal lig.
21 Longissimus cervicis
22 Deep cervical v.
23 Longissimus capitis & splenius cervicis
24 Trapezius
25 Splenius capitis
26 Semispinalis capitis
27 Semispinalis cervicis
28 Lig. flavum
29 Spinal cord
30 CERV. VERT. IV

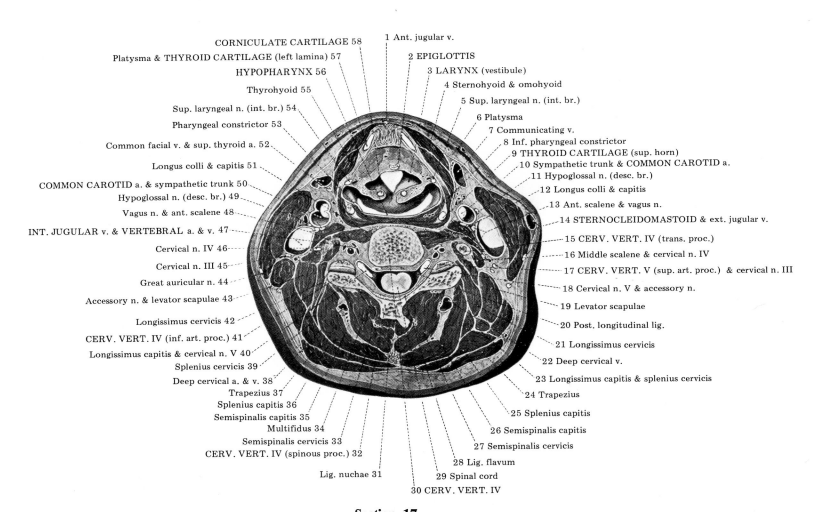

Section 17

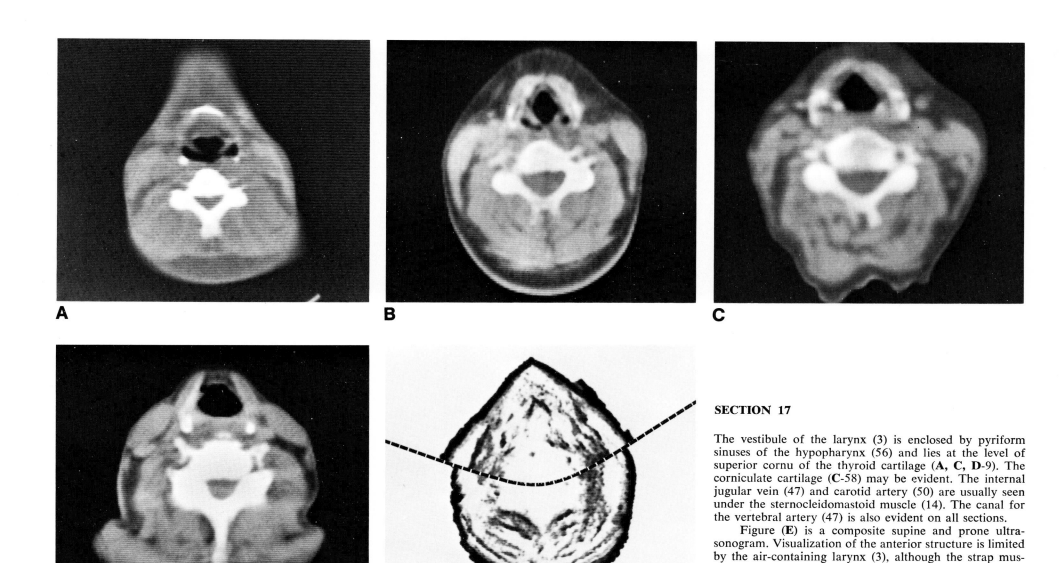

A

B

C

D

E

SECTION 17

The vestibule of the larynx (3) is enclosed by pyriform sinuses of the hypopharynx (56) and lies at the level of superior cornu of the thyroid cartilage (**A, C, D**-9). The corniculate cartilage (**C**-58) may be evident. The internal jugular vein (47) and carotid artery (50) are usually seen under the sternocleidomastoid muscle (14). The canal for the vertebral artery (47) is also evident on all sections.

Figure (**E**) is a composite supine and prone ultrasonogram. Visualization of the anterior structure is limited by the air-containing larynx (3), although the strap muscles of the neck are evident anteriorly. The sternocleidomastoid (14) and a jugular vein (47) are again seen. Posteriorly there is visualization of the neck muscles and the spinous process of a cervical vertebra.

KEY FIGURES V, VI, VII, VIII These key figures cover not only the trunk but also the lower neck, upper arms, and upper legs. The pelvis, which includes the pelvic cavity, genitalia, buttocks, and anus, is also covered in the following sections. The levels of the sections are indicated by the transverse lines in the following key figures.

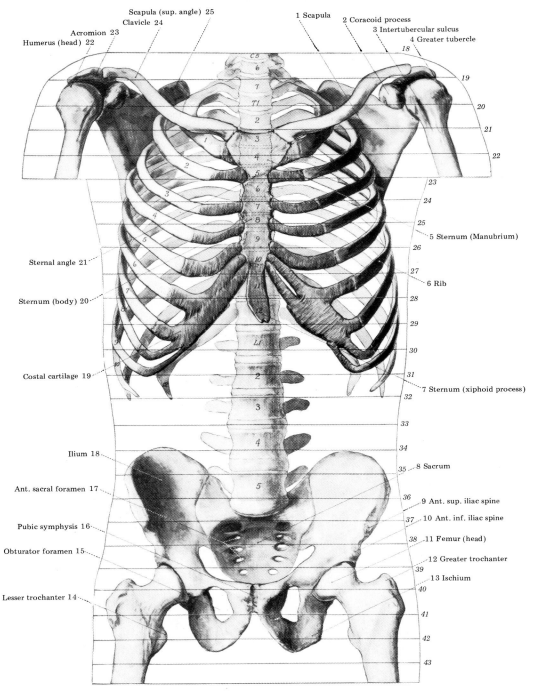

Scapula (sup. angle) 25
Clavicle 24
Acromion 23
Humerus (head) 22

1 Scapula
2 Coracoid process
3 Intertubercular sulcus
4 Greater tubercle

18
19
20
21
22
23
24
25

5 Sternum (Manubrium)

26
27

6 Rib

28
29
30
31

7 Sternum (xiphoid process)

32
33
34
35

8 Sacrum

Sternal angle 21
Sternum (body) 20
Costal cartilage 19
Ilium 18
Ant. sacral foramen 17
Pubic symphysis 16
Obturator foramen 15
Lesser trochanter 14

36
37
38
39
40
41
42
43

9 Ant. sup. iliac spine
10 Ant. inf. iliac spine
11 Femur (head)
12 Greater trochanter
13 Ischium

KEY FIGURE V   This represents a front view of the skeleton of the
trunk showing the levels of the sections through the bones.

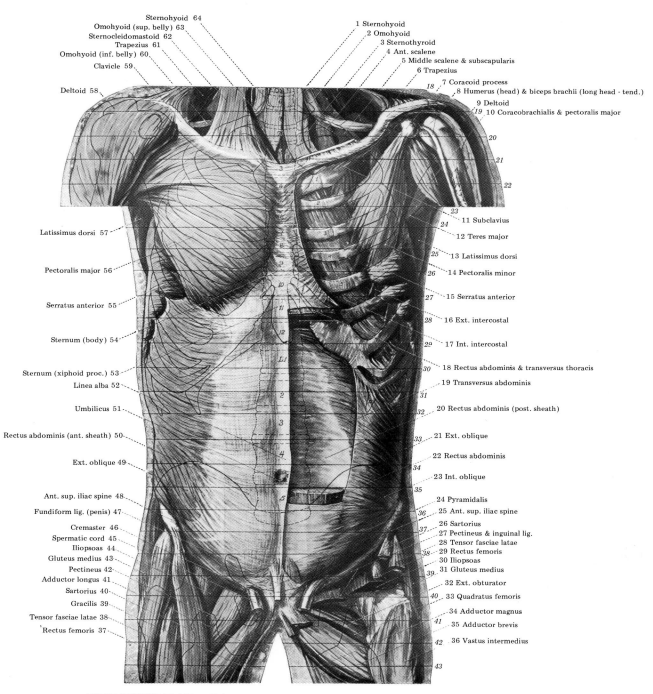

Sternohyoid 64
Omohyoid (sup. belly) 63
Sternocleidomastoid 62
Trapezius 61
Omohyoid (inf. belly) 60
Clavicle 59

Deltoid 58

Latissimus dorsi 57

Pectoralis major 56

Serratus anterior 55

Sternum (body) 54

Sternum (xiphoid proc.) 53
Linea alba 52

Umbilicus 51

Rectus abdominis (ant. sheath) 50

Ext. oblique 49

Ant. sup. iliac spine 48
Fundiform lig. (penis) 47
Cremaster 46
Spermatic cord 45
Iliopsoas 44
Gluteus medius 43
Pectineus 42
Adductor longus 41
Sartorius 40
Gracilis 39
Tensor fasciae latae 38
Rectus femoris 37

1 Sternohyoid
2 Omohyoid
3 Sternothyroid
4 Ant. scalene
5 Middle scalene & subscapularis
6 Trapezius
18 7 Coracoid process
8 Humerus (head) & biceps brachii (long head - tend.)
9 Deltoid
19 10 Coracobrachialis & pectoralis major
20
21
22
23
24 11 Subclavius
12 Teres major
25 13 Latissimus dorsi
26 14 Pectoralis minor
27 15 Serratus anterior
28 16 Ext. intercostal
29 17 Int. intercostal
30 18 Rectus abdominis & transversus thoracis
19 Transversus abdominis
31
32 20 Rectus abdominis (post. sheath)
33 21 Ext. oblique
22 Rectus abdominis
34
23 Int. oblique
35
24 Pyramidalis
36 25 Ant. sup. iliac spine
26 Sartorius
37 27 Pectineus & inguinal lig.
28 Tensor fasciae latae
38 29 Rectus femoris
30 Iliopsoas
39 31 Gluteus medius
32 Ext. obturator
40 33 Quadratus femoris
34 Adductor magnus
41 35 Adductor brevis
42 36 Vastus intermedius
43

KEY FIGURE VI   This represents a front view of the muscles of
the trunk with an outline of the skeleton indicated by black lines. Note
that certain muscles have been removed on the left side to show the
underlying muscles.

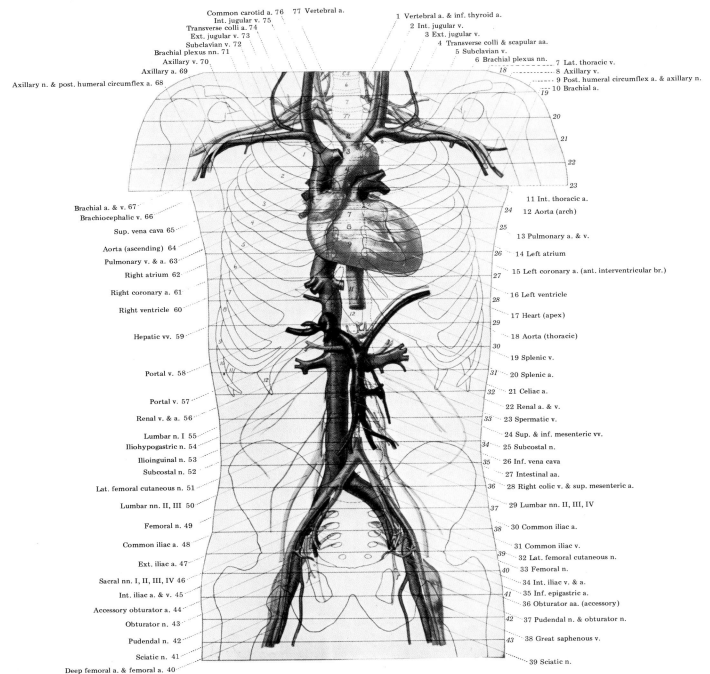

Common carotid a. 76   77 Vertebral a.
Int. jugular v. 75
Transverse colli a. 74
Ext. jugular v. 73
Subclavian v. 72
Brachial plexus nn. 71
Axillary v. 70
Axillary a. 69
Axillary n. & post. humeral circumflex a. 68

1 Vertebral a. & inf. thyroid a.
2 Int. jugular v.
3 Ext. jugular v.
4 Transverse colli & scapular aa.
5 Subclavian v.
6 Brachial plexus nn.
7 Lat. thoracic v.
8 Axillary v.
9 Post. humeral circumflex a. & axillary n.
10 Brachial a.

Brachial a. & v. 67
Brachiocephalic v. 66
Sup. vena cava 65
Aorta (ascending) 64
Pulmonary v. & a. 63
Right atrium 62
Right coronary a. 61
Right ventricle 60
Hepatic vv. 59
Portal v. 58
Portal v. 57
Renal v. & a. 56
Lumbar n. I 55
Iliohypogastric n. 54
Ilioinguinal n. 53
Subcostal n. 52
Lat. femoral cutaneous n. 51
Lumbar nn. II, III 50
Femoral n. 49
Common iliac a. 48
Ext. iliac a. 47
Sacral nn. I, II, III, IV 46
Int. iliac a. & v. 45
Accessory obturator a. 44
Obturator n. 43
Pudendal n. 42
Sciatic n. 41
Deep femoral a. & femoral a. 40

11 Int. thoracic a.
12 Aorta (arch)
13 Pulmonary a. & v.
14 Left atrium
15 Left coronary a. (ant. interventricular br.)
16 Left ventricle
17 Heart (apex)
18 Aorta (thoracic)
19 Splenic v.
20 Splenic a.
21 Celiac a.
22 Renal a. & v.
23 Spermatic v.
24 Sup. & inf. mesenteric vv.
25 Subcostal n.
26 Inf. vena cava
27 Intestinal aa.
28 Right colic v. & sup. mesenteric a.
29 Lumbar nn. II, III, IV
30 Common iliac a.
31 Common iliac v.
32 Lat. femoral cutaneous n.
33 Femoral n.
34 Int. iliac v. & a.
35 Inf. epigastric a.
36 Obturator aa. (accessory)
37 Pudendal n. & obturator n.
38 Great saphenous v.
39 Sciatic n.

KEY FIGURE VII This represents a front view of the heart, the principal blood vessels as well as the spinal nerve trunks and plexuses.

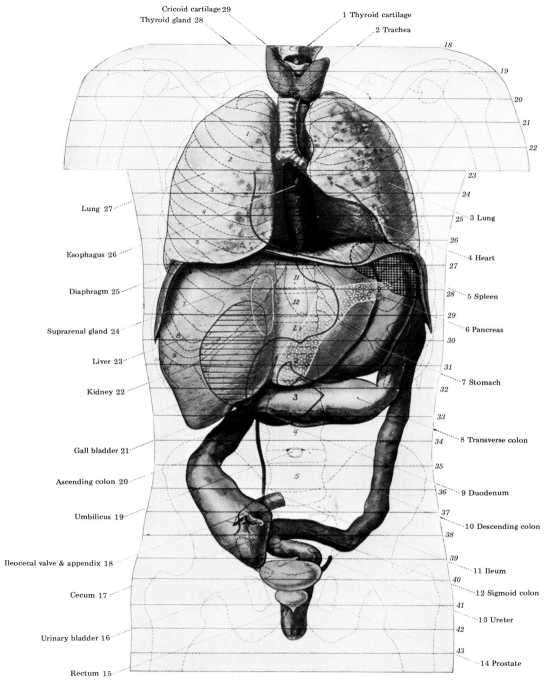

Cricoid cartilage 29
Thyroid gland 28
1 Thyroid cartilage
2 Trachea

Lung 27

Esophagus 26

Diaphragm 25

Suprarenal gland 24

Liver 23

Kidney 22

Gall bladder 21

Ascending colon 20

Umbilicus 19

Ileocecal valve & appendix 18

Cecum 17

Urinary bladder 16

Rectum 15

18
19
20
21
22
23
24
25 3 Lung
26
27 4 Heart
28 5 Spleen
29
30 6 Pancreas
31
32 7 Stomach
33
34 8 Transverse colon
35
36 9 Duodenum
37
38 10 Descending colon
39
40 11 Ileum
41 12 Sigmoid colon
42 13 Ureter
43 14 Prostate

KEY FIGURE VIII This shows the topography of the thoracic and abdominal viscera.

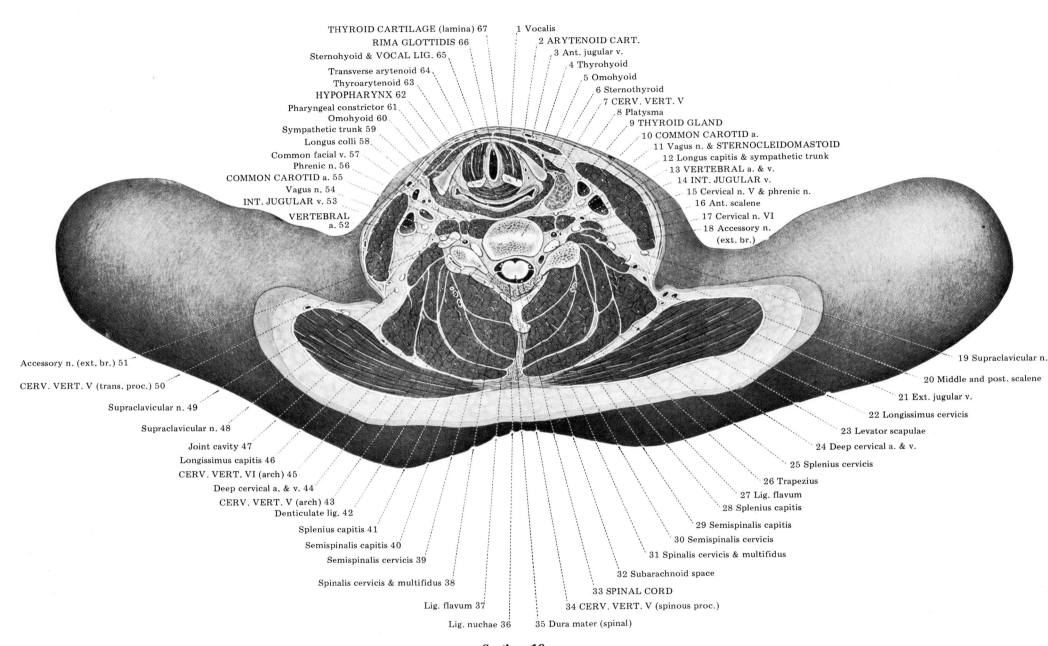

THYROID CARTILAGE (lamina) 67
RIMA GLOTTIDIS 66
Sternohyoid & VOCAL LIG. 65
Transverse arytenoid 64
Thyroarytenoid 63
HYPOPHARYNX 62
Pharyngeal constrictor 61
Omohyoid 60
Sympathetic trunk 59
Longus colli 58
Common facial v. 57
Phrenic n. 56
COMMON CAROTID a. 55
Vagus n. 54
INT. JUGULAR v. 53
VERTEBRAL
a. 52

1 Vocalis
2 ARYTENOID CART.
3 Ant. jugular v.
4 Thyrohyoid
5 Omohyoid
6 Sternothyroid
7 CERV. VERT. V
8 Platysma
9 THYROID GLAND
10 COMMON CAROTID a.
11 Vagus n. & STERNOCLEIDOMASTOID
12 Longus capitis & sympathetic trunk
13 VERTEBRAL a. & v.
14 INT. JUGULAR v.
15 Cervical n. V & phrenic n.
16 Ant. scalene
17 Cervical n. VI
18 Accessory n.
(ext. br.)

Accessory n. (ext. br.) 51
CERV. VERT. V (trans. proc.) 50
Supraclavicular n. 49
Supraclavicular n. 48
Joint cavity 47
Longissimus capitis 46
CERV. VERT. VI (arch) 45
Deep cervical a. & v. 44
CERV. VERT. V (arch) 43
Denticulate lig. 42
Splenius capitis 41
Semispinalis capitis 40
Semispinalis cervicis 39
Spinalis cervicis & multifidus 38
Lig. flavum 37
Lig. nuchae 36

19 Supraclavicular n.
20 Middle and post. scalene
21 Ext. jugular v.
22 Longissimus cervicis
23 Levator scapulae
24 Deep cervical a. & v.
25 Splenius cervicis
26 Trapezius
27 Lig. flavum
28 Splenius capitis
29 Semispinalis capitis
30 Semispinalis cervicis
31 Spinalis cervicis & multifidus
32 Subarachnoid space
33 SPINAL CORD
34 CERV. VERT. V (spinous proc.)
35 Dura mater (spinal)

Section 18

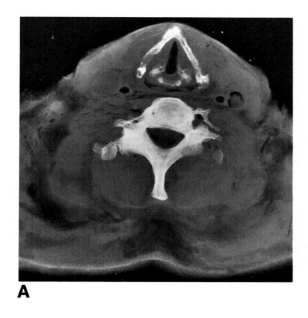

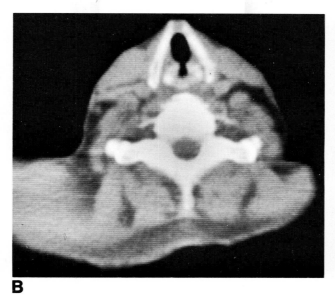

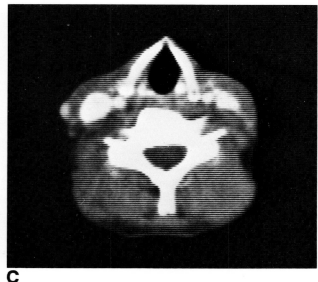

A

B

C

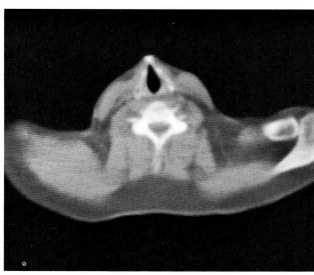

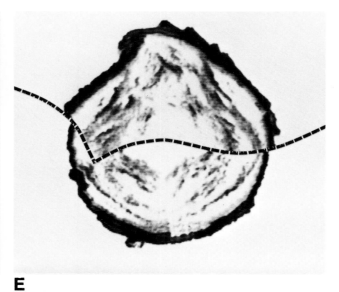

D

E

SECTION 18

At the level of the vocal cords, the glottis (66) is enclosed by thyroid cartilage (67) and arytenoid cartilages (2). The common carotid artery (55) and internal jugular vein (53) lie under the sternocleidomastoid muscle (11), and they are filled with air on the specimen (**A**) and with contrast during rapid intravenous infusion on the scan (**C**). The external jugular vein may also be seen lying subcutaneously (cf. Section 17 [14]).

Figure (**E**) is a composite ultrasonogram from supine and prone films. The larynx limits the visualization of anterior structures. The sternocleidomastoid muscles (11) are now larger, and located more anteriorly. The jugular veins (53) can be easily defined. The posterior muscles are thinner and flatter with the trapezius muscle (26) appearing quite prominent. The spine is more anteriorly situated.

Section 18

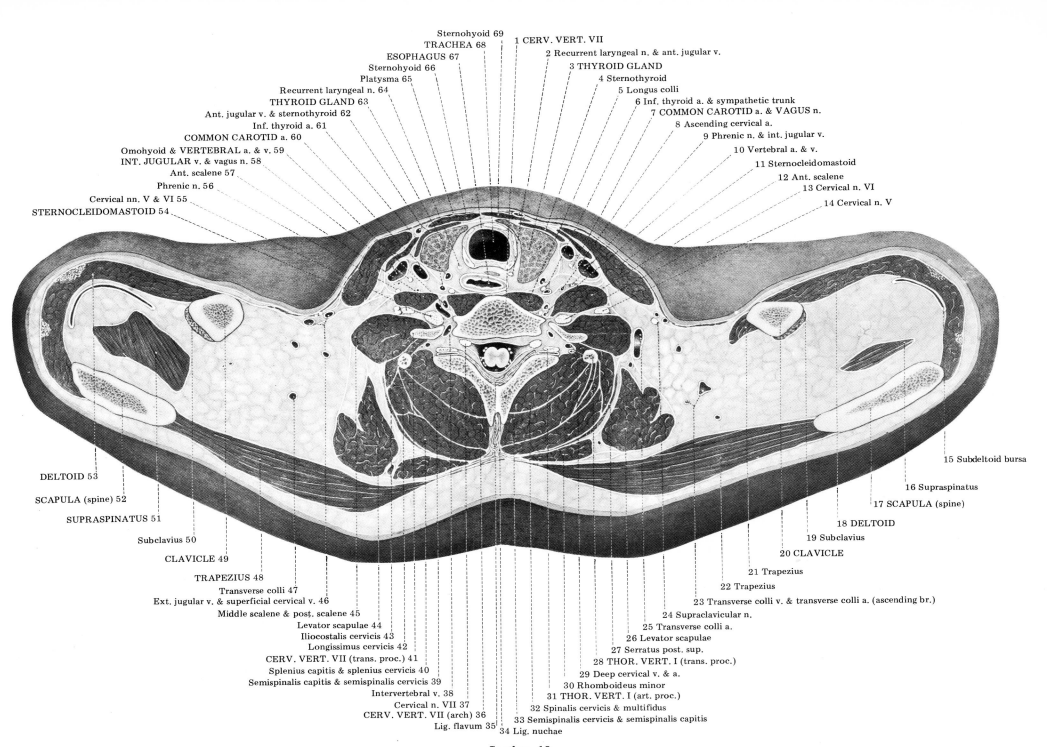

Sternohyoid 69
TRACHEA 68
ESOPHAGUS 67
Sternohyoid 66
Platysma 65
Recurrent laryngeal n. 64
THYROID GLAND 63
Ant. jugular v. & sternothyroid 62
Inf. thyroid a. 61
COMMON CAROTID a. 60
Omohyoid & VERTEBRAL a. & v. 59
INT. JUGULAR v. & vagus n. 58
Ant. scalene 57
Phrenic n. 56
Cervical nn. V & VI 55
STERNOCLEIDOMASTOID 54

1 CERV. VERT. VII
2 Recurrent laryngeal n. & ant. jugular v.
3 THYROID GLAND
4 Sternothyroid
5 Longus colli
6 Inf. thyroid a. & sympathetic trunk
7 COMMON CAROTID a. & VAGUS n.
8 Ascending cervical a.
9 Phrenic n. & int. jugular v.
10 Vertebral a. & v.
11 Sternocleidomastoid
12 Ant. scalene
13 Cervical n. VI
14 Cervical n. V

15 Subdeltoid bursa
16 Supraspinatus
17 SCAPULA (spine)
18 DELTOID
19 Subclavius
20 CLAVICLE
21 Trapezius
22 Trapezius
23 Transverse colli v. & transverse colli a. (ascending br.)
24 Supraclavicular n.
25 Transverse colli a.
26 Levator scapulae
27 Serratus post. sup.
28 THOR. VERT. I (trans. proc.)
29 Deep cervical v. & a.
30 Rhomboideus minor
31 THOR. VERT. I (art. proc.)
32 Spinalis cervicis & multifidus
33 Semispinalis cervicis & semispinalis capitis
34 Lig. nuchae

DELTOID 53
SCAPULA (spine) 52
SUPRASPINATUS 51
Subclavius 50
CLAVICLE 49
TRAPEZIUS 48
Transverse colli 47
Ext. jugular v. & superficial cervical v. 46
Middle scalene & post. scalene 45
Levator scapulae 44
Iliocostalis cervicis 43
Longissimus cervicis 42
CERV. VERT. VII (trans. proc.) 41
Splenius capitis & splenius cervicis 40
Semispinalis capitis & semispinalis cervicis 39
Intervertebral v. 38
Cervical n. VII 37
CERV. VERT. VII (arch) 36
Lig. flavum 35
34 Lig. nuchae

Section 19

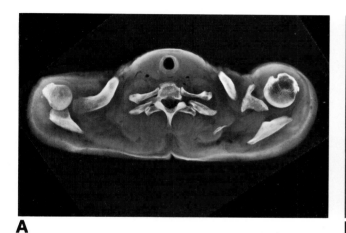

A

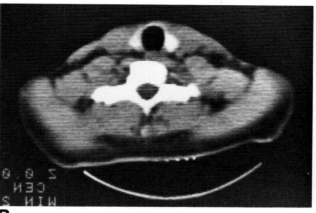

B

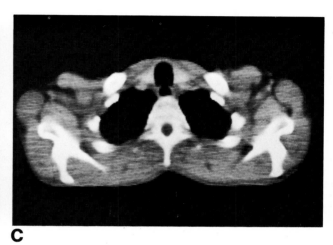

C

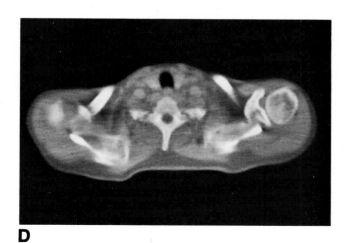

D

SECTION 19

Immediately below or caudad to the thyroid cartilage is the thyroid gland (3). This gland is well seen on a plain CT scan because of its high iodine content. Note the flat or concave configuration of the posterior wall of the trachea (68) adjacent to the esophagus (67). The carotid artery (60) and jugular vein (58) are outlined by air in the specimen (**A**) and lie under the sternocleidomastoid muscle (54). Also note the anterior scalene muscle (12), distal clavicle (20), scapula (17), and humeral head with biceps groove (**A, E**-cf. Section 20[19]).

Section 19

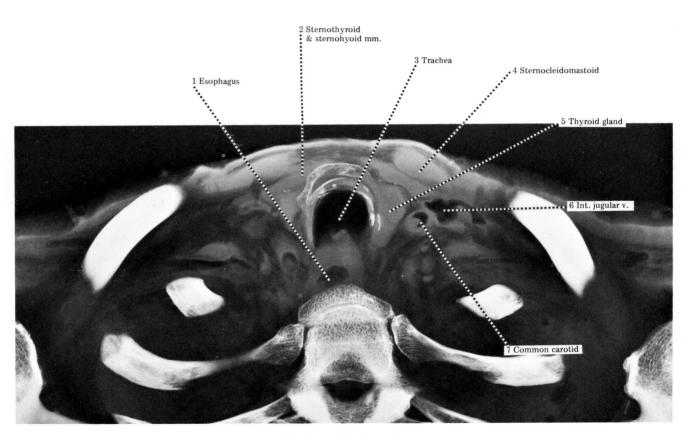

1 Esophagus

2 Sternothyroid
& sternohyoid mm.

3 Trachea

4 Sternocleidomastoid

5 Thyroid gland

6 Int. jugular v.

7 Common carotid

Section 19   (x-ray)

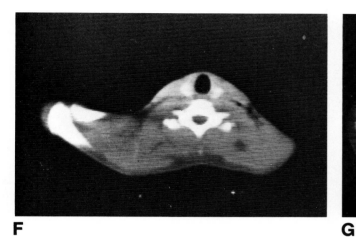

F

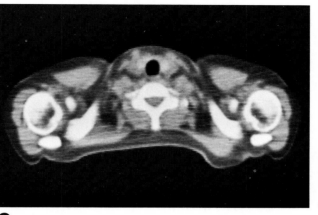

G

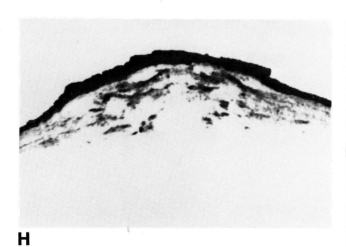

H

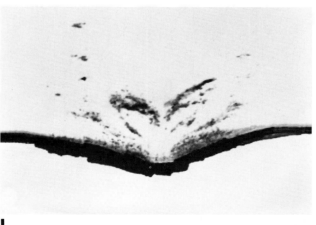

I

SECTION 19 (cont.)

A second specimen (left) and two other CT scans (**F**) and (**G**), also at the level of the thyroid gland (5), show some of the variations in appearance of this structure and of the muscles and vessels that lie in the area.

The thyroid gland (5) forms a major part of the anterior transonic shadow (**H**). The tracheal air column is poorly demonstrated behind it. The major neck vessels are seen with some difficulty posterolateral to the thyroid gland. Posteriorly (**I**) the trapezius muscle now presents as a major structure, and the remaining lower neck muscles are also clearly defined.

Echographic sections of the thorax below this level present very little useful information because of the thin soft tissues, ribs, and underlying lungs. Therefore, no ultrasonic images are presented for Sections 20 through 27.

Section 19

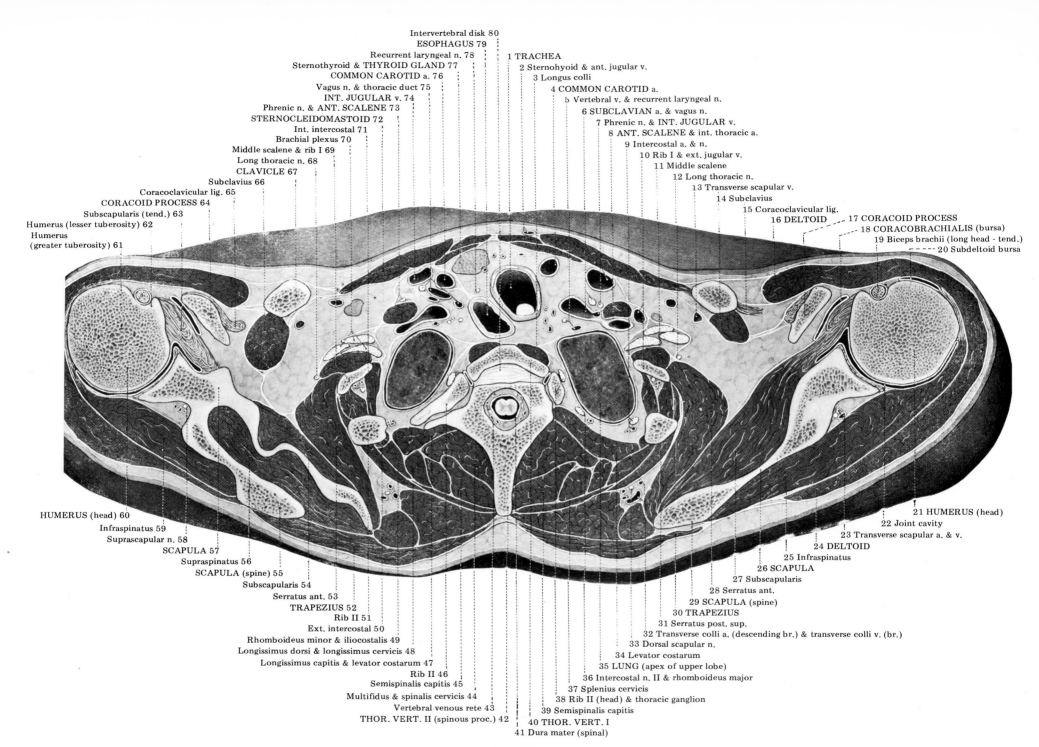

Intervertebral disk 80
ESOPHAGUS 79
Recurrent laryngeal n. 78
Sternothyroid & THYROID GLAND 77
COMMON CAROTID a. 76
Vagus n. & thoracic duct 75
INT. JUGULAR v. 74
Phrenic n. & ANT. SCALENE 73
STERNOCLEIDOMASTOID 72
Int. intercostal 71
Brachial plexus 70
Middle scalene & rib I 69
Long thoracic n. 68
CLAVICLE 67
Subclavius 66
Coracoclavicular lig. 65
CORACOID PROCESS 64
Subscapularis (tend.) 63
Humerus (lesser tuberosity) 62
Humerus
(greater tuberosity) 61

1 TRACHEA
2 Sternohyoid & ant. jugular v.
3 Longus colli
4 COMMON CAROTID a.
5 Vertebral v. & recurrent laryngeal n.
6 SUBCLAVIAN a. & vagus n.
7 Phrenic n. & INT. JUGULAR v.
8 ANT. SCALENE & int. thoracic a.
9 Intercostal a. & n.
10 Rib I & ext. jugular v.
11 Middle scalene
12 Long thoracic n.
13 Transverse scapular v.
14 Subclavius
15 Coracoclavicular lig.
16 DELTOID — 17 CORACOID PROCESS
18 CORACOBRACHIALIS (bursa)
19 Biceps brachii (long head - tend.)
20 Subdeltoid bursa

HUMERUS (head) 60
Infraspinatus 59
Suprascapular n. 58
SCAPULA 57
Supraspinatus 56
SCAPULA (spine) 55
Subscapularis 54
Serratus ant. 53
TRAPEZIUS 52
Rib II 51
Ext. intercostal 50
Rhomboideus minor & iliocostalis 49
Longissimus dorsi & longissimus cervicis 48
Longissimus capitis & levator costarum 47
Rib II 46
Semispinalis capitis 45
Multifidus & spinalis cervicis 44
Vertebral venous rete 43
THOR. VERT. II (spinous proc.) 42

21 HUMERUS (head)
22 Joint cavity
23 Transverse scapular a. & v.
24 DELTOID
25 Infraspinatus
26 SCAPULA
27 Subscapularis
28 Serratus ant.
29 SCAPULA (spine)
30 TRAPEZIUS
31 Serratus post. sup.
32 Transverse colli a. (descending br.) & transverse colli v. (br.)
33 Dorsal scapular n.
34 Levator costarum
35 LUNG (apex of upper lobe)
36 Intercostal n. II & rhomboideus major
37 Splenius cervicis
38 Rib II (head) & thoracic ganglion
39 Semispinalis capitis
40 THOR. VERT. I
41 Dura mater (spinal)

Section 20

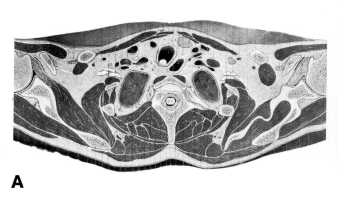

A

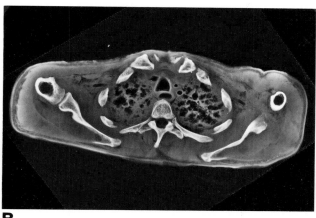

B

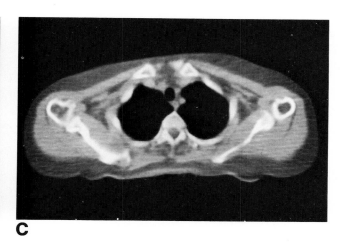

C

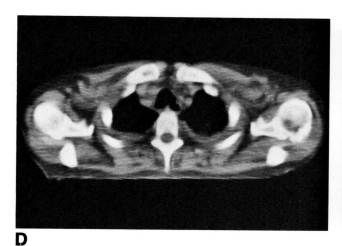

D

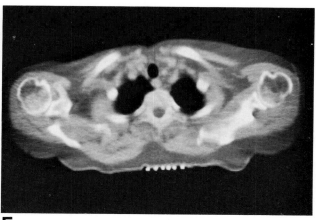

E

SECTION 20

Figure (**A**) is Section 20 reversed. The brachiocephalic vessels are seen with the subclavian artery (6) lying posterolateral to the trachea (1), whereas the carotid artery (76) and internal jugular vein (74) lie anterolaterally. The arteries are outlined by air on the specimen (**B**). The esophagus (79) is behind or to the left of the trachea and contains air (**B**) and (**D**). These sections show the mid- or proximal clavicle, scapula (25), glenoid fossa (22), and head of humerus (21). Note the bicipital groove (19), deltoid (16), infraspinatus (25), and subscapularis (27) muscles. The apices of the lungs (35), ribs, and thoracic spine are also evident, as is the coracoid process (**E**-64).

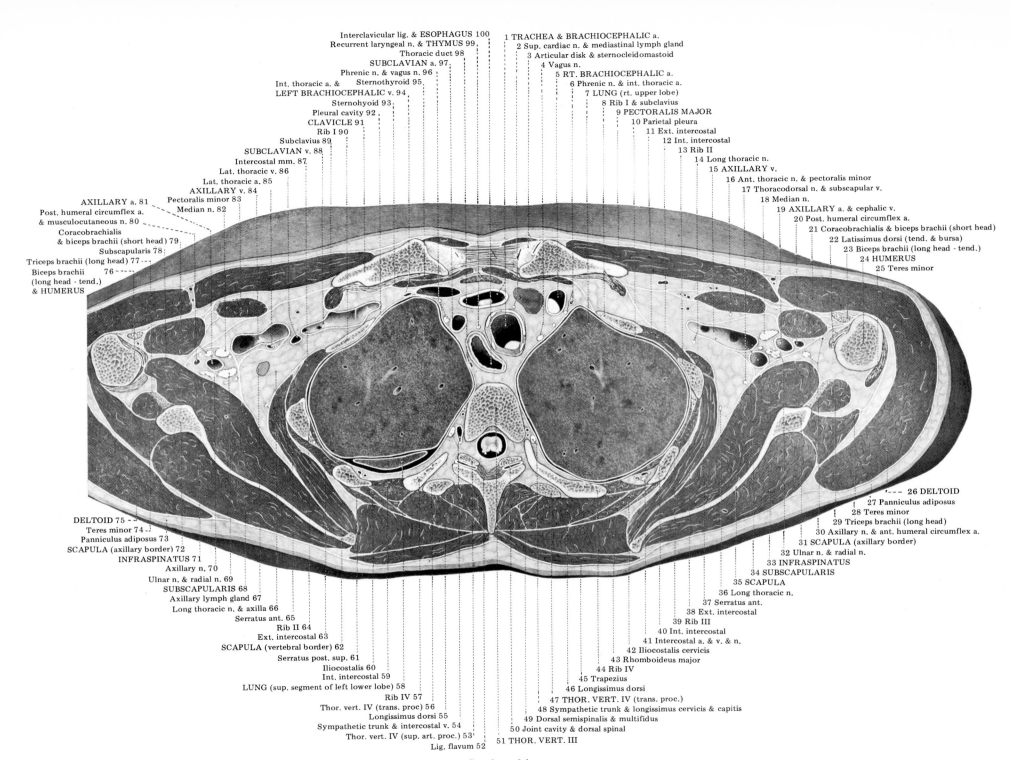

Interclavicular lig. & ESOPHAGUS 100
Recurrent laryngeal n. & THYMUS 99
Thoracic duct 98
SUBCLAVIAN a. 97
Phrenic n. & vagus n. 96
Int. thoracic a. &　Sternothyroid 95
LEFT BRACHIOCEPHALIC v. 94
Sternohyoid 93
Pleural cavity 92
CLAVICLE 91
Rib I 90
Subclavius 89
SUBCLAVIAN v. 88
Intercostal mm. 87
Lat. thoracic v. 86
Lat. thoracic a. 85
AXILLARY v. 84
Pectoralis minor 83
AXILLARY a. 81　Median n. 82
Post. humeral circumflex a.
& musculocutaneous n. 80
Coracobrachialis
& biceps brachii (short head) 79
Subscapularis 78
Triceps brachii (long head) 77
Biceps brachii
(long head - tend.)
76
& HUMERUS

1 TRACHEA & BRACHIOCEPHALIC a.
2 Sup. cardiac n. & mediastinal lymph gland
3 Articular disk & sternocleidomastoid
4 Vagus n.
5 RT. BRACHIOCEPHALIC a.
6 Phrenic n. & int. thoracic a.
7 LUNG (rt. upper lobe)
8 Rib I & subclavius
9 PECTORALIS MAJOR
10 Parietal pleura
11 Ext. intercostal
12 Int. intercostal
13 Rib II
14 Long thoracic n.
15 AXILLARY v.
16 Ant. thoracic n. & pectoralis minor
17 Thoracodorsal n. & subscapular v.
18 Median n.
19 AXILLARY a. & cephalic v.
20 Post. humeral circumflex a.
21 Coracobrachialis & biceps brachii (short head)
22 Latissimus dorsi (tend. & bursa)
23 Biceps brachii (long head - tend.)
24 HUMERUS
25 Teres minor

26 DELTOID
27 Panniculus adiposus
28 Teres minor
29 Triceps brachii (long head)
30 Axillary n. & ant. humeral circumflex a.
31 SCAPULA (axillary border)
32 Ulnar n. & radial n.
33 INFRASPINATUS
34 SUBSCAPULARIS
35 SCAPULA
36 Long thoracic n.
37 Serratus ant.
38 Ext. intercostal
39 Rib III
40 Int. intercostal
41 Intercostal a. & v. & n.
42 Iliocostalis cervicis
43 Rhomboideus major
44 Rib IV
45 Trapezius
46 Longissimus dorsi
47 THOR. VERT. IV (trans. proc.)
48 Sympathetic trunk & longissimus cervicis & capitis
49 Dorsal semispinalis & multifidus
50 Joint cavity & dorsal spinal
51 THOR. VERT. III

DELTOID 75
Teres minor 74
Panniculus adiposus 73
SCAPULA (axillary border) 72
INFRASPINATUS 71
Axillary n. 70
Ulnar n. & radial n. 69
SUBSCAPULARIS 68
Axillary lymph gland 67
Long thoracic n. & axilla 66
Serratus ant. 65
Rib II 64
Ext. intercostal 63
SCAPULA (vertebral border) 62
Serratus post. sup. 61
Iliocostalis 60
Int. intercostal 59
LUNG (sup. segment of left lower lobe) 58
Rib IV 57
Thor. vert. IV (trans. proc) 56
Longissimus dorsi 55
Sympathetic trunk & intercostal v. 54
Thor. vert. IV (sup. art. proc.) 53
Lig. flavum 52

Section 21

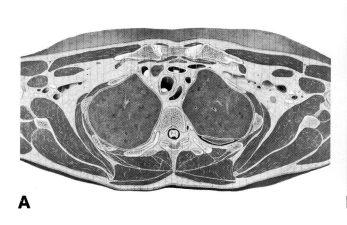

A

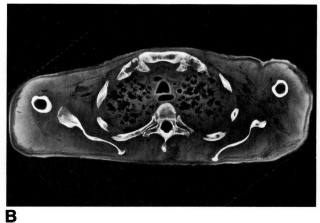

B

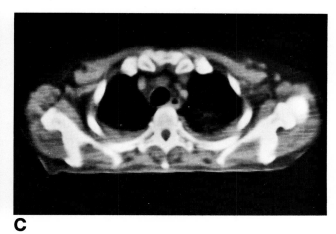

C

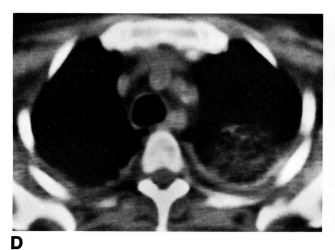

D

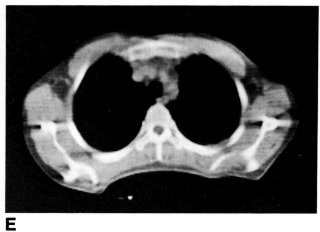

E

SECTION 21

Figure (**A**) is Section 21 reversed. The innominate artery (1) lies anterior to the trachea (1), whereas the left subclavian artery (97) and left common carotid artery lie laterally. These vessels are outlined by air on the specimen (**B**). The brachiocephalic veins (5, 94) are behind the heads of the clavicles (91). The esophagus (100) is seen posterolateral to the trachea on the left and contains air as seen in Figures (**B**) and (**C**). The scapulae (35), thoracic spine (51), ribs (39), manubrium sternum, and sternoclavicular joints are also evident. Pulmonary edema and pleural effusions are present in (**B**), (**C**), and (**D**).

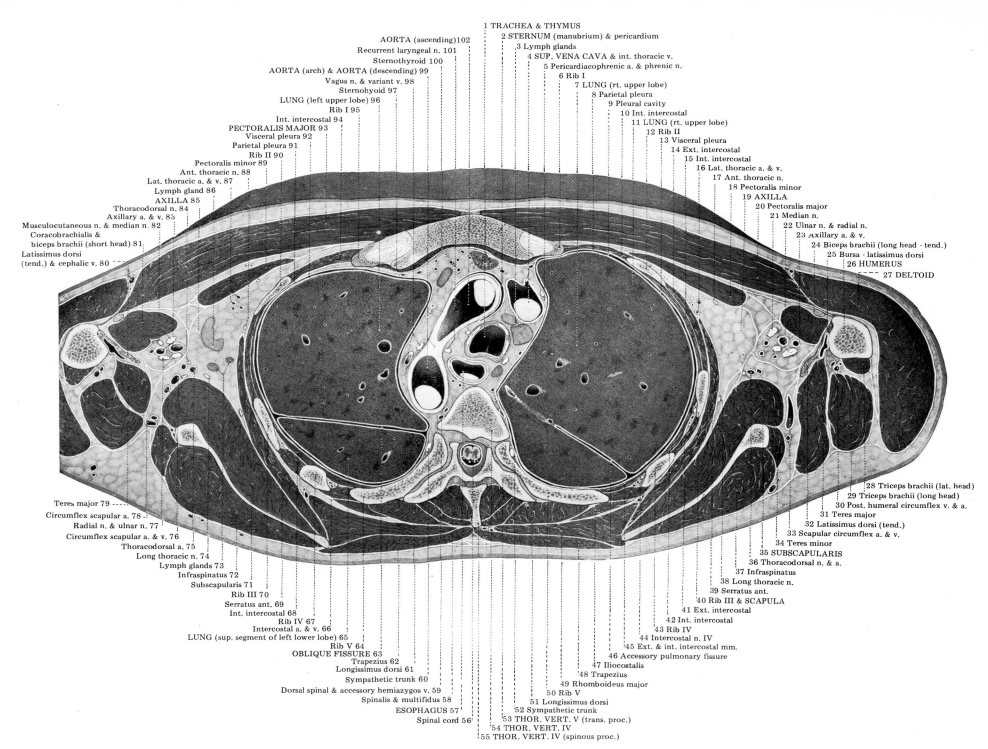

1 TRACHEA & THYMUS
AORTA (ascending)102
2 STERNUM (manubrium) & pericardium
Recurrent laryngeal n. 101
3 Lymph glands
Sternothyroid 100
4 SUP. VENA CAVA & int. thoracic v.
AORTA (arch) & AORTA (descending) 99
5 Pericardiacophrenic a. & phrenic n.
Vagus n. & variant v. 98
6 Rib I
Sternohyoid 97
7 LUNG (rt. upper lobe)
LUNG (left upper lobe) 96
8 Parietal pleura
Rib I 95
9 Pleural cavity
Int. intercostal 94
10 Int. intercostal
PECTORALIS MAJOR 93
11 LUNG (rt. upper lobe)
Visceral pleura 92
12 Rib II
Parietal pleura 91
13 Visceral pleura
Rib II 90
14 Ext. intercostal
Pectoralis minor 89
15 Int. intercostal
Ant. thoracic n. 88
16 Lat. thoracic a. & v.
Lat. thoracic a. & v. 87
17 Ant. thoracic n.
Lymph gland 86
18 Pectoralis minor
AXILLA 85
19 AXILLA
Thoracodorsal n. 84
20 Pectoralis major
Axillary a. & v. 83
21 Median n.
Musculocutaneous n. & median n. 82
22 Ulnar n. & radial n.
Coracobrachialis &
23 Axillary a. & v.
biceps brachii (short head) 81
24 Biceps brachii (long head - tend.)
25 Bursa - latissimus dorsi
Latissimus dorsi
26 HUMERUS
(tend.) & cephalic v. 80
27 DELTOID

28 Triceps brachii (lat. head)
29 Triceps brachii (long head)
Teres major 79
30 Post. humeral circumflex v. & a.
Circumflex scapular a. 78
31 Teres major
Radial n. & ulnar n. 77
32 Latissimus dorsi (tend.)
Circumflex scapular a. & v. 76
33 Scapular circumflex a. & v.
Thoracodorsal a. 75
34 Teres minor
Long thoracic n. 74
35 SUBSCAPULARIS
Lymph glands 73
36 Thoracodorsal n. & a.
Infraspinatus 72
37 Infraspinatus
Subscapularis 71
38 Long thoracic n.
Rib III 70
39 Serratus ant.
Serratus ant. 69
40 Rib III & SCAPULA
Int. intercostal 68
41 Ext. intercostal
Rib IV 67
42 Int. intercostal
Intercostal a. & v. 66
43 Rib IV
LUNG (sup. segment of left lower lobe) 65
44 Intercostal n. IV
Rib V 64
45 Ext. & int. intercostal mm.
OBLIQUE FISSURE 63
46 Accessory pulmonary fissure
Trapezius 62
47 Iliocostalis
Longissimus dorsi 61
48 Trapezius
Sympathetic trunk 60
49 Rhomboideus major
Dorsal spinal & accessory hemiazygos v. 59
50 Rib V
Spinalis & multifidus 58
51 Longissimus dorsi
ESOPHAGUS 57
52 Sympathetic trunk
Spinal cord 56
53 THOR. VERT. V (trans. proc.)
54 THOR. VERT. IV
55 THOR. VERT. IV (spinous proc.)

Section 22

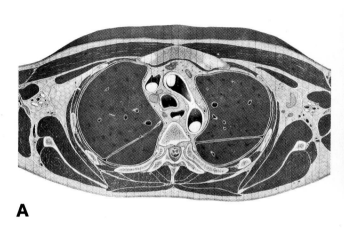

A

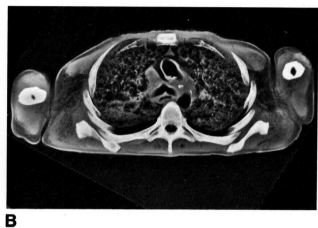

B

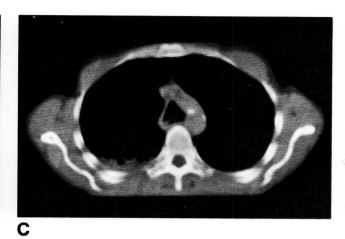

C

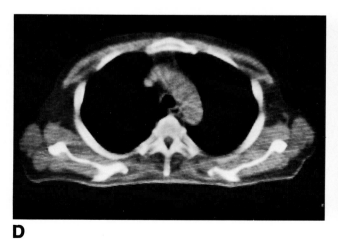

D

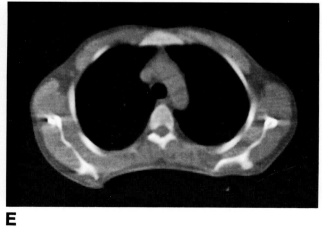

E

SECTION 22

Figure (**A**) is Section 22 reversed. The aortic arch can be seen anterior and to the left of the trachea (1) and esophagus (57). A CT scan (**C**) of a cadaver corresponding to (**B**) is at the level of the carina, whereas scans (**D**) and (**E**) are taken at slightly higher levels in two patients. Note that the superior vena cava (4) lies to the right of the ascending aorta (102). There is a variation in the appearance of the anterior mediastinum. The manubrium (2), scapulae (40), ribs (40), thoracic spine (54), and humeri (**B**-26) are well seen.

Section 22

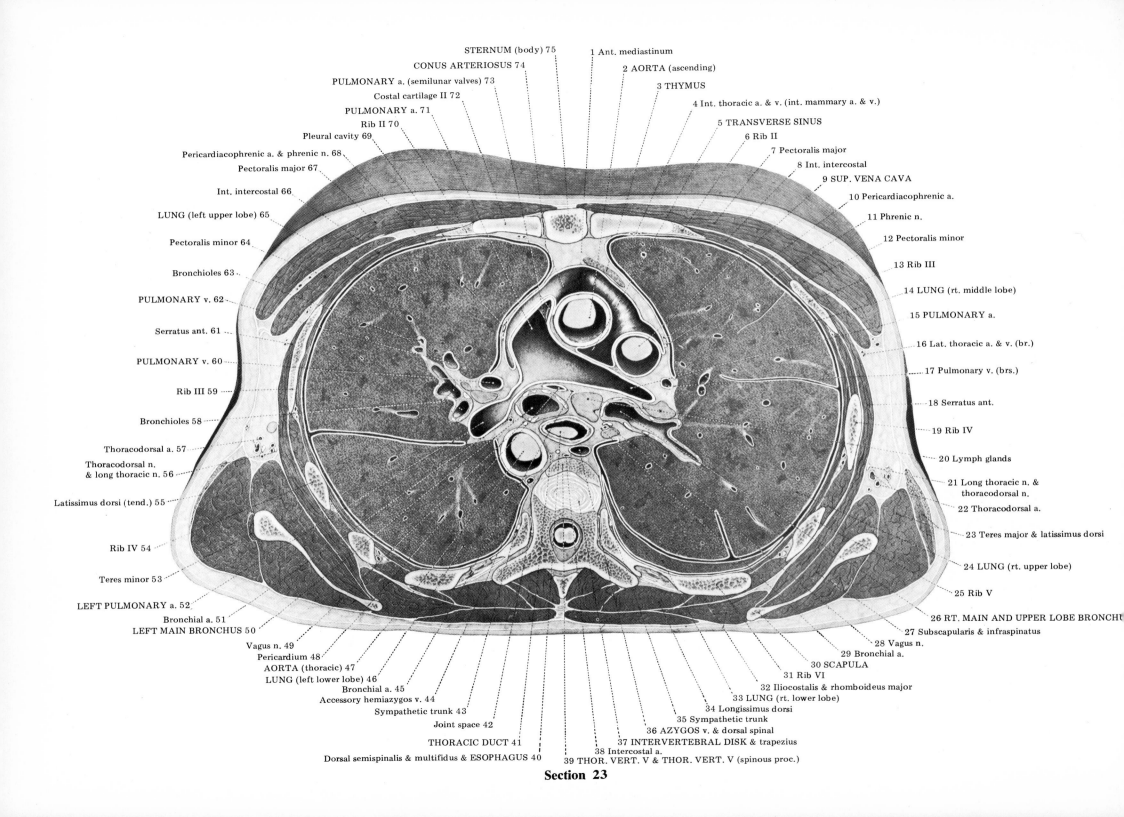

STERNUM (body) 75
1 Ant. mediastinum
CONUS ARTERIOSUS 74
2 AORTA (ascending)
PULMONARY a. (semilunar valves) 73
3 THYMUS
Costal cartilage II 72
4 Int. thoracic a. & v. (int. mammary a. & v.)
PULMONARY a. 71
5 TRANSVERSE SINUS
Rib II 70
6 Rib II
Pleural cavity 69
7 Pectoralis major
Pericardiacophrenic a. & phrenic n. 68
8 Int. intercostal
Pectoralis major 67
9 SUP. VENA CAVA
Int. intercostal 66
10 Pericardiacophrenic a.
LUNG (left upper lobe) 65
11 Phrenic n.
Pectoralis minor 64
12 Pectoralis minor
Bronchioles 63
13 Rib III
PULMONARY v. 62
14 LUNG (rt. middle lobe)
15 PULMONARY a.
Serratus ant. 61
16 Lat. thoracic a. & v. (br.)
PULMONARY v. 60
17 Pulmonary v. (brs.)
Rib III 59
18 Serratus ant.
Bronchioles 58
19 Rib IV
Thoracodorsal a. 57
20 Lymph glands
Thoracodorsal n. & long thoracic n. 56
21 Long thoracic n. & thoracodorsal n.
22 Thoracodorsal a.
Latissimus dorsi (tend.) 55
23 Teres major & latissimus dorsi
24 LUNG (rt. upper lobe)
Rib IV 54
25 Rib V
Teres minor 53
26 RT. MAIN AND UPPER LOBE BRONCHU
LEFT PULMONARY a. 52
27 Subscapularis & infraspinatus
Bronchial a. 51
28 Vagus n.
LEFT MAIN BRONCHUS 50
29 Bronchial a.
Vagus n. 49
30 SCAPULA
Pericardium 48
31 Rib VI
AORTA (thoracic) 47
32 Iliocostalis & rhomboideus major
LUNG (left lower lobe) 46
33 LUNG (rt. lower lobe)
Bronchial a. 45
34 Longissimus dorsi
Accessory hemiazygos v. 44
35 Sympathetic trunk
Sympathetic trunk 43
36 AZYGOS v. & dorsal spinal
Joint space 42
37 INTERVERTEBRAL DISK & trapezius
THORACIC DUCT 41
38 Intercostal a.
39 THOR. VERT. V & THOR. VERT. V (spinous proc.)
Dorsal semispinalis & multifidus & ESOPHAGUS 40

Section 23

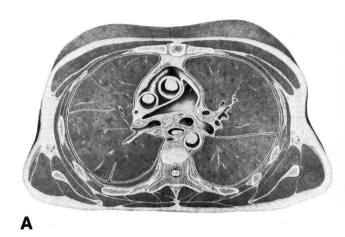

A

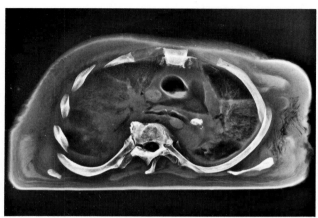

B

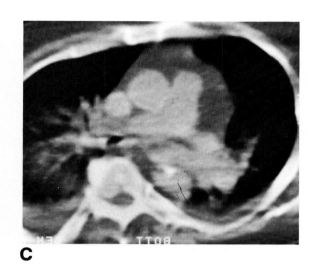

C

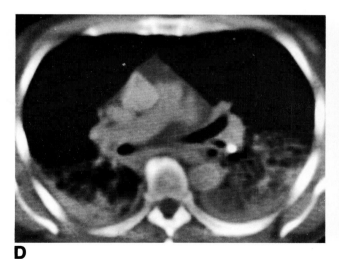

D

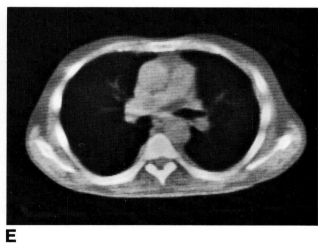

E

SECTION 23

Figure (**A**) is Section 23 reversed. An x-ray of a specimen (**B**) and the corresponding scan (**C**) taken of a cadaver are just below the carina. Scans (**D**) of a second cadaver and (**E**) from a patient show the right bronchus intermedius just caudad to the upper lobe bronchus (26) and left main bronchus (50) at the same level as the right (15) and left (52) pulmonary arteries. The main pulmonary artery (71) is to the left of the ascending aorta (2). The superior vena cava (9) lies anterior to the right pulmonary artery. The descending aorta (47) is to the left of the thoracic spine (39). The azygos vein (36) lies just anterior to the spine (39) and behind the esophagus (40). The internal mammary vessels (**E**-4) may be visualized when the window has been adjusted for the pulmonary vessels. Pulmonary edema and pleural effusions are present in the cadavers (**B**), (**C**), and (**D**).

Section 23

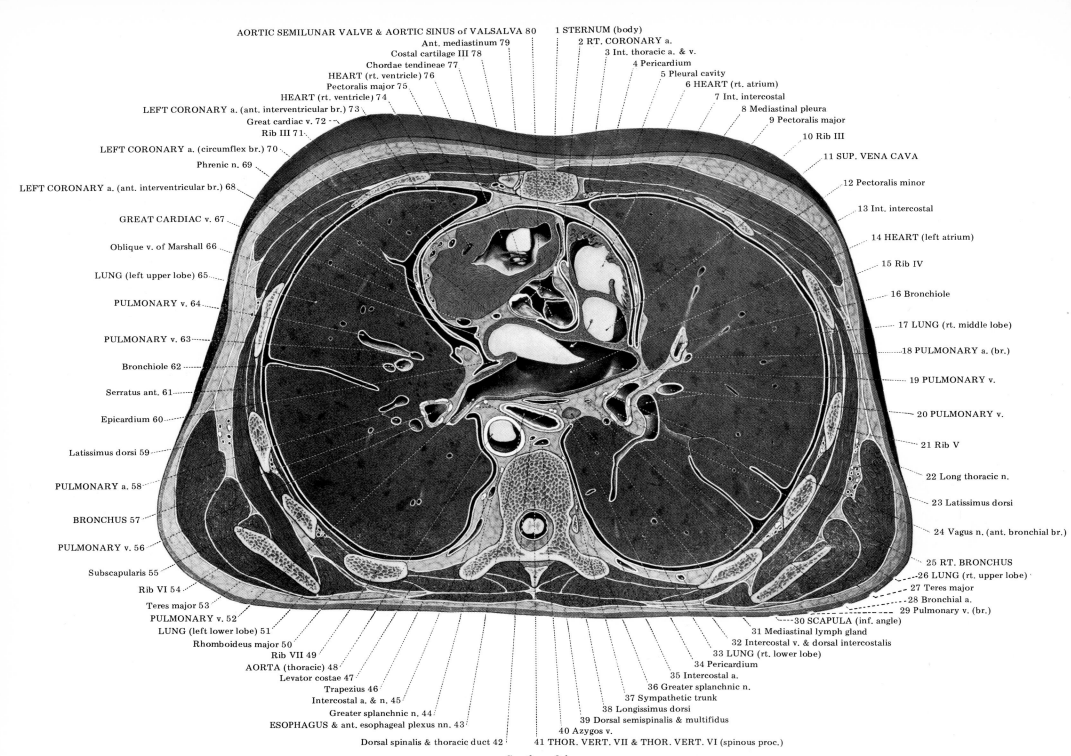

AORTIC SEMILUNAR VALVE & AORTIC SINUS of VALSALVA 80
Ant. mediastinum 79
Costal cartilage III 78
Chordae tendineae 77
HEART (rt. ventricle) 76
Pectoralis major 75
HEART (rt. ventricle) 74
LEFT CORONARY a. (ant. interventricular br.) 73
Great cardiac v. 72
Rib III 71
LEFT CORONARY a. (circumflex br.) 70
Phrenic n. 69
LEFT CORONARY a. (ant. interventricular br.) 68
GREAT CARDIAC v. 67
Oblique v. of Marshall 66
LUNG (left upper lobe) 65
PULMONARY v. 64
PULMONARY v. 63
Bronchiole 62
Serratus ant. 61
Epicardium 60
Latissimus dorsi 59
PULMONARY a. 58
BRONCHUS 57
PULMONARY v. 56
Subscapularis 55
Rib VI 54
Teres major 53
PULMONARY v. 52
LUNG (left lower lobe) 51
Rhomboideus major 50
Rib VII 49
AORTA (thoracic) 48
Levator costae 47
Trapezius 46
Intercostal a. & n. 45
Greater splanchnic n. 44
ESOPHAGUS & ant. esophageal plexus nn. 43
Dorsal spinalis & thoracic duct 42

1 STERNUM (body)
2 RT. CORONARY a.
3 Int. thoracic a. & v.
4 Pericardium
5 Pleural cavity
6 HEART (rt. atrium)
7 Int. intercostal
8 Mediastinal pleura
9 Pectoralis major
10 Rib III
11 SUP. VENA CAVA
12 Pectoralis minor
13 Int. intercostal
14 HEART (left atrium)
15 Rib IV
16 Bronchiole
17 LUNG (rt. middle lobe)
18 PULMONARY a. (br.)
19 PULMONARY v.
20 PULMONARY v.
21 Rib V
22 Long thoracic n.
23 Latissimus dorsi
24 Vagus n. (ant. bronchial br.)
25 RT. BRONCHUS
26 LUNG (rt. upper lobe)
27 Teres major
28 Bronchial a.
29 Pulmonary v. (br.)
30 SCAPULA (inf. angle)
31 Mediastinal lymph gland
32 Intercostal v. & dorsal intercostalis
33 LUNG (rt. lower lobe)
34 Pericardium
35 Intercostal a.
36 Greater splanchnic n.
37 Sympathetic trunk
38 Longissimus dorsi
39 Dorsal semispinalis & multifidus
40 Azygos v.
41 THOR. VERT. VII & THOR. VERT. VI (spinous proc.)

Section 24

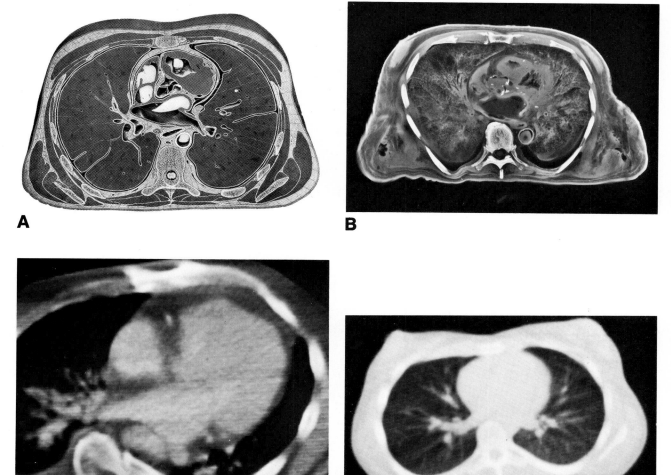

A

B

C

D

E

SECTION 24

Figure (**A**) is Section 24 reversed. The right (19) and left (52) pulmonary veins, which are caudad to the pulmonary arteries (cf. Section 23) and carina, drain into the left atrium (14). The right atrium (6), superior vena cava (11), aortic valve (80), and right ventricle (76) are discernible. The right middle lobe (17) and lingular segment of the left upper lobe (65) may be separated anteriorly only by the pleura (**C**-79) under the sternum (1). The descending aorta (48) lies to the left of the spine (41). The right (25) and left (57) bronchi are visible within the hilar areas. The CT scan (**C**) is from the same cadaver and level as the specimen (**B**), and scan (**D**) is of another cadaver. Scan (**E**) is of a patient with a window adjusted for visualization of the pulmonary vessels. The cardiac chambers may be visible even with a scan time of 2.5 minutes. Pleural effusions due to congestive heart failure are present in both cadavers (**C**) and (**D**).

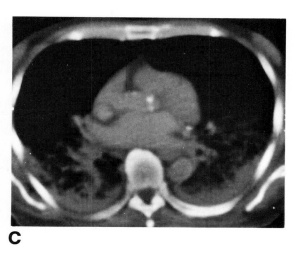

Section 24

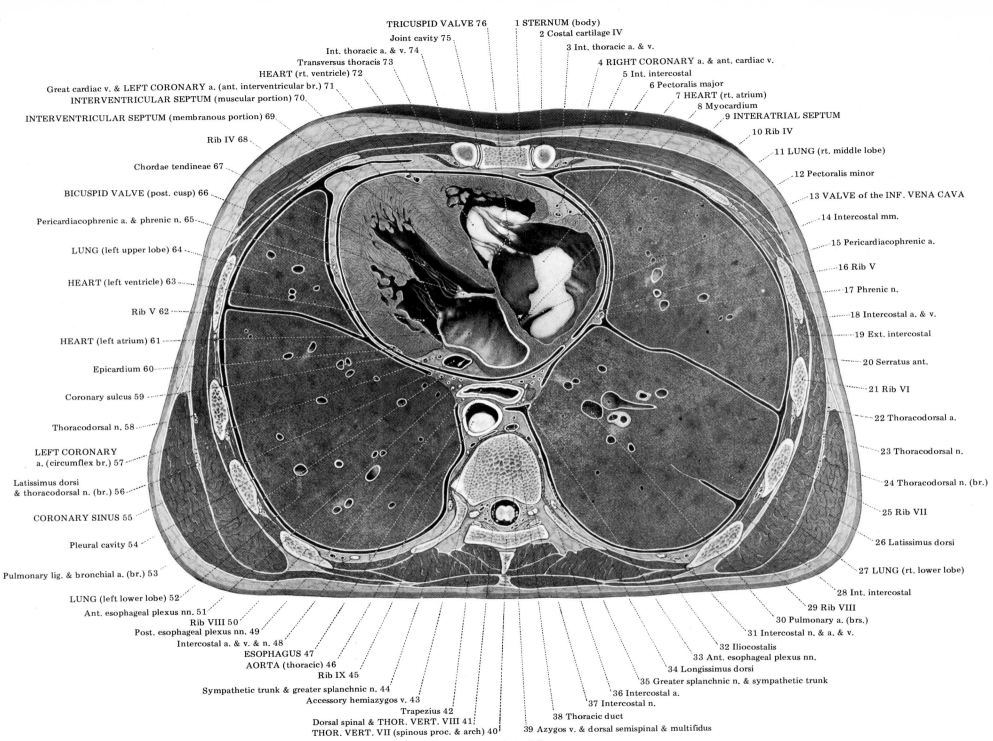

TRICUSPID VALVE 76
1 STERNUM (body)
Joint cavity 75
2 Costal cartilage IV
Int. thoracic a. & v. 74
3 Int. thoracic a. & v.
Transversus thoracis 73
4 RIGHT CORONARY a. & ant. cardiac v.
HEART (rt. ventricle) 72
5 Int. intercostal
6 Pectoralis major
Great cardiac v. & LEFT CORONARY a. (ant. interventricular br.) 71
7 HEART (rt. atrium)
INTERVENTRICULAR SEPTUM (muscular portion) 70
8 Myocardium
INTERVENTRICULAR SEPTUM (membranous portion) 69
9 INTERATRIAL SEPTUM
10 Rib IV
Rib IV 68
11 LUNG (rt. middle lobe)
Chordae tendineae 67
12 Pectoralis minor
BICUSPID VALVE (post. cusp) 66
13 VALVE of the INF. VENA CAVA
Pericardiacophrenic a. & phrenic n. 65
14 Intercostal mm.
15 Pericardiacophrenic a.
LUNG (left upper lobe) 64
16 Rib V
HEART (left ventricle) 63
17 Phrenic n.
18 Intercostal a. & v.
Rib V 62
19 Ext. intercostal
HEART (left atrium) 61
20 Serratus ant.
Epicardium 60
21 Rib VI
Coronary sulcus 59
22 Thoracodorsal a.
Thoracodorsal n. 58
23 Thoracodorsal n.
LEFT CORONARY
a. (circumflex br.) 57
24 Thoracodorsal n. (br.)
Latissimus dorsi
& thoracodorsal n. (br.) 56
25 Rib VII
CORONARY SINUS 55
26 Latissimus dorsi
Pleural cavity 54
27 LUNG (rt. lower lobe)
Pulmonary lig. & bronchial a. (br.) 53
28 Int. intercostal
29 Rib VIII
LUNG (left lower lobe) 52
30 Pulmonary a. (brs.)
Ant. esophageal plexus nn. 51
31 Intercostal n. & a. & v.
Rib VIII 50
32 Iliocostalis
Post. esophageal plexus nn. 49
33 Ant. esophageal plexus nn.
Intercostal a. & v. & n. 48
34 Longissimus dorsi
ESOPHAGUS 47
35 Greater splanchnic n. & sympathetic trunk
AORTA (thoracic) 46
36 Intercostal a.
Rib IX 45
37 Intercostal n.
Sympathetic trunk & greater splanchnic n. 44
38 Thoracic duct
Accessory hemiazygos v. 43
39 Azygos v. & dorsal semispinal & multifidus
Trapezius 42
Dorsal spinal & THOR. VERT. VIII 41
THOR. VERT. VII (spinous proc. & arch) 40

Section 25

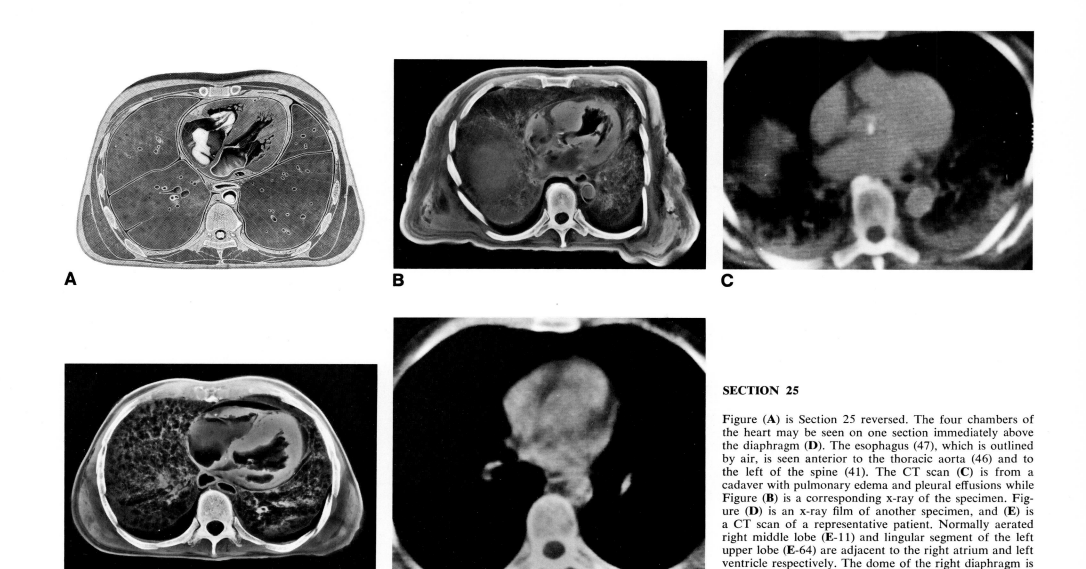

A

B

C

D

E

SECTION 25

Figure (**A**) is Section 25 reversed. The four chambers of the heart may be seen on one section immediately above the diaphragm (**D**). The esophagus (47), which is outlined by air, is seen anterior to the thoracic aorta (46) and to the left of the spine (41). The CT scan (**C**) is from a cadaver with pulmonary edema and pleural effusions while Figure (**B**) is a corresponding x-ray of the specimen. Figure (**D**) is an x-ray film of another specimen, and (**E**) is a CT scan of a representative patient. Normally aerated right middle lobe (**E**-11) and lingular segment of the left upper lobe (**E**-64) are adjacent to the right atrium and left ventricle respectively. The dome of the right diaphragm is visible in Figures (**B**) and (**C**).

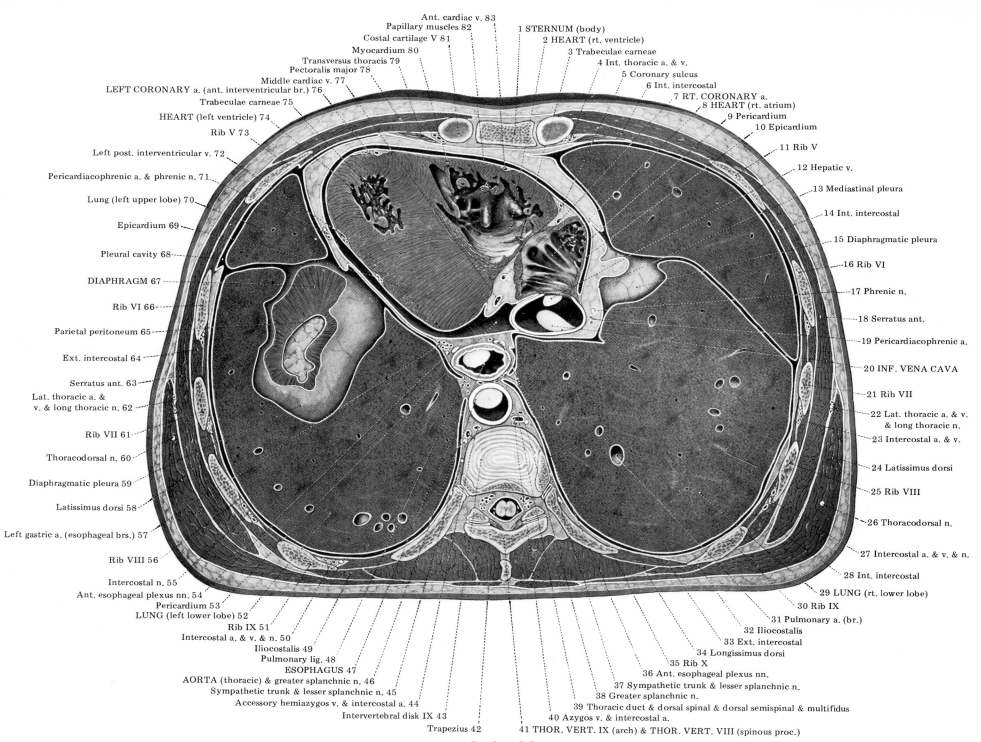

Ant. cardiac v. 83
Papillary muscles 82
Costal cartilage V 81
Myocardium 80
Transversus thoracis 79
Pectoralis major 78
Middle cardiac v. 77
LEFT CORONARY a. (ant. interventricular br.) 76
Trabeculae carneae 75
HEART (left ventricle) 74
Rib V 73
Left post. interventricular v. 72
Pericardiacophrenic a. & phrenic n. 71
Lung (left upper lobe) 70
Epicardium 69
Pleural cavity 68
DIAPHRAGM 67
Rib VI 66
Parietal peritoneum 65
Ext. intercostal 64
Serratus ant. 63
Lat. thoracic a. & v. & long thoracic n. 62
Rib VII 61
Thoracodorsal n. 60
Diaphragmatic pleura 59
Latissimus dorsi 58
Left gastric a. (esophageal brs.) 57
Rib VIII 56
Intercostal n. 55
Ant. esophageal plexus nn. 54
Pericardium 53
LUNG (left lower lobe) 52
Rib IX 51
Intercostal a. & v. & n. 50
Iliocostalis 49
Pulmonary lig. 48
ESOPHAGUS 47
AORTA (thoracic) & greater splanchnic n. 46
Sympathetic trunk & lesser splanchnic n. 45
Accessory hemiazygos v. & intercostal a. 44
Intervertebral disk IX 43
Trapezius 42

1 STERNUM (body)
2 HEART (rt. ventricle)
3 Trabeculae carneae
4 Int. thoracic a. & v.
5 Coronary sulcus
6 Int. intercostal
7 RT. CORONARY a.
8 HEART (rt. atrium)
9 Pericardium
10 Epicardium
11 Rib V
12 Hepatic v.
13 Mediastinal pleura
14 Int. intercostal
15 Diaphragmatic pleura
16 Rib VI
17 Phrenic n.
18 Serratus ant.
19 Pericardiacophrenic a.
20 INF. VENA CAVA
21 Rib VII
22 Lat. thoracic a. & v. & long thoracic n.
23 Intercostal a. & v.
24 Latissimus dorsi
25 Rib VIII
26 Thoracodorsal n.
27 Intercostal a. & v. & n.
28 Int. intercostal
29 LUNG (rt. lower lobe)
30 Rib IX
31 Pulmonary a. (br.)
32 Iliocostalis
33 Ext. intercostal
34 Longissimus dorsi
35 Rib X
36 Ant. esophageal plexus nn.
37 Sympathetic trunk & lesser splanchnic n.
38 Greater splanchnic n.
39 Thoracic duct & dorsal spinal & dorsal semispinal & multifidus
40 Azygos v. & intercostal a.
41 THOR. VERT. IX (arch) & THOR. VERT. VIII (spinous proc.)

Section 26

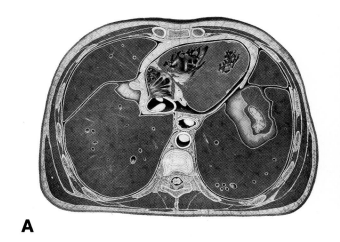

A

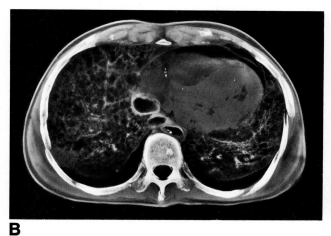

B

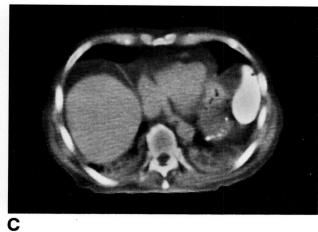

C

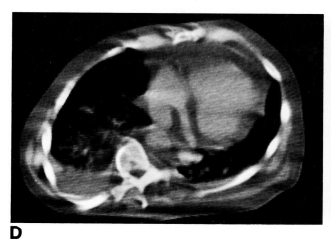

D

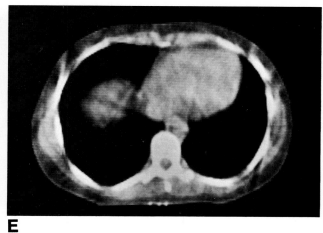

E

SECTION 26

Figure (**A**) is Section 26 reversed. Figure (**B**) is an x-ray of a specimen, (**C**) and (**D**) are scans of cadavers, and (**E**) is a scan of a patient. The most inferior section of the heart shows the inferior vena cava (20) entering the right atrium (8), which is separated from the right (2) and left (74) ventricles by the coronary sulcus (5). Fat in the epicardium (10) and surrounding the coronary vessels (76) may be discernible. The esophagus (47) lies between the thoracic aorta (46) and inferior vena cava (20). The dome of diaphragm (**C**-15, **C**-67, **E**-15) is visible. Barium is seen within the splenic flexure of the colon (**C**). The deformity of the thoracic cage in (**D**) is due to scoliosis. Pulmonary edema in the lower lobes (29) and pleural effusions are evident in both cadavers (**C**) and (**D**).

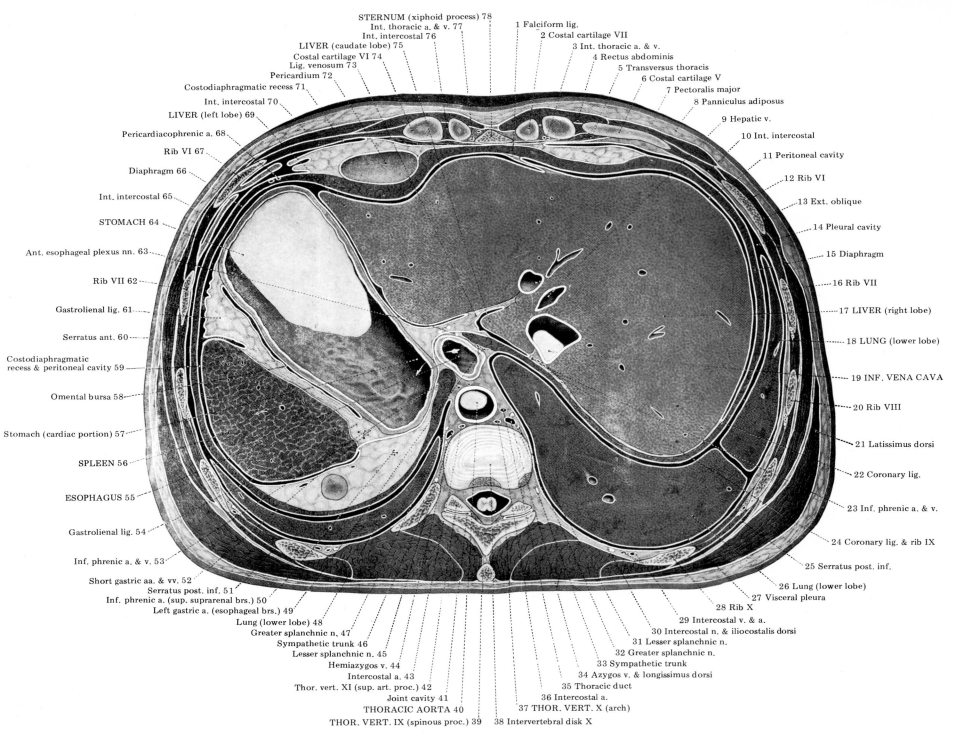

STERNUM (xiphoid process) 78
Int. thoracic a. & v. 77
Int. intercostal 76
LIVER (caudate lobe) 75
Costal cartilage VI 74
Lig. venosum 73
Pericardium 72
Costodiaphragmatic recess 71
Int. intercostal 70
LIVER (left lobe) 69
Pericardiacophrenic a. 68
Rib VI 67
Diaphragm 66
Int. intercostal 65
STOMACH 64
Ant. esophageal plexus nn. 63
Rib VII 62
Gastrolienal lig. 61
Serratus ant. 60
Costodiaphragmatic recess & peritoneal cavity 59
Omental bursa 58
Stomach (cardiac portion) 57
SPLEEN 56
ESOPHAGUS 55
Gastrolienal lig. 54
Inf. phrenic a. & v. 53
Short gastric aa. & vv. 52
Serratus post. inf. 51
Inf. phrenic a. (sup. suprarenal brs.) 50
Left gastric a. (esophageal brs.) 49
Lung (lower lobe) 48
Greater splanchnic n. 47
Sympathetic trunk 46
Lesser splanchnic n. 45
Hemiazygos v. 44
Intercostal a. 43
Thor. vert. XI (sup. art. proc.) 42
Joint cavity 41
THORACIC AORTA 40
THOR. VERT. IX (spinous proc.) 39

1 Falciform lig.
2 Costal cartilage VII
3 Int. thoracic a. & v.
4 Rectus abdominis
5 Transversus thoracis
6 Costal cartilage V
7 Pectoralis major
8 Panniculus adiposus
9 Hepatic v.
10 Int. intercostal
11 Peritoneal cavity
12 Rib VI
13 Ext. oblique
14 Pleural cavity
15 Diaphragm
16 Rib VII
17 LIVER (right lobe)
18 LUNG (lower lobe)
19 INF. VENA CAVA
20 Rib VIII
21 Latissimus dorsi
22 Coronary lig.
23 Inf. phrenic a. & v.
24 Coronary lig. & rib IX
25 Serratus post. inf.
26 Lung (lower lobe)
27 Visceral pleura
28 Rib X
29 Intercostal v. & a.
30 Intercostal n. & iliocostalis dorsi
31 Lesser splanchnic n.
32 Greater splanchnic n.
33 Sympathetic trunk
34 Azygos v. & longissimus dorsi
35 Thoracic duct
36 Intercostal a.
37 THOR. VERT. X (arch)
38 Intervertebral disk X

Section 27

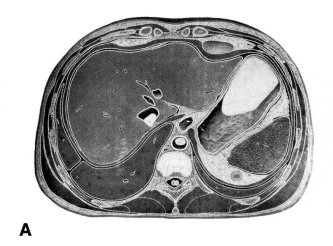

A

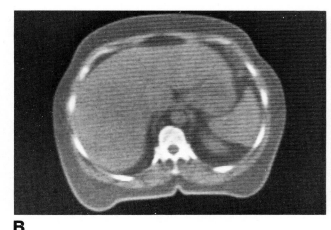

B

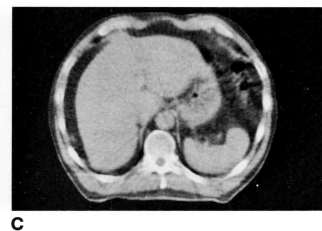

C

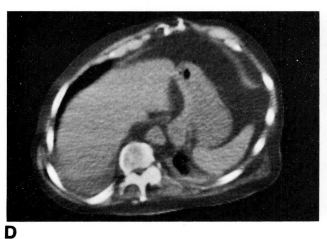

D

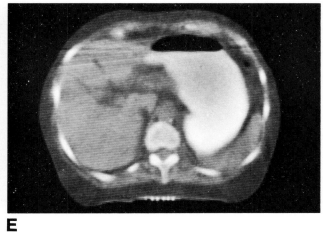

E

SECTION 27

Figure (**A**) is Section 27 reversed. The aorta (40), which is encompassed by the diaphragm, spleen (56), and liver (17, 69, 75), can be seen at this level; all vary in appearance between patients. The vena cava (19) is immediately behind the caudate lobe of the liver (75) which is separated from the left lobe (69) by the ligamentum venosum (73). The right lobe of the liver (17) may be partially outlined by fat (**C**) or by the lower lobe of the lung (**D**-18). The stomach (64) which contains fluid and air (**B, C, D**) has been outlined with dilute Gastrografin * in Figure (**E**). Normal bile ducts may be seen within the liver and are easily seen when dilated. Note azygos (**C**-34) and hemiazygos (**C**-44) veins.

* Meglumine diatrizoate (66%) and sodium diatrizoate (10%) oral solution, E. R. Squibb & Sons

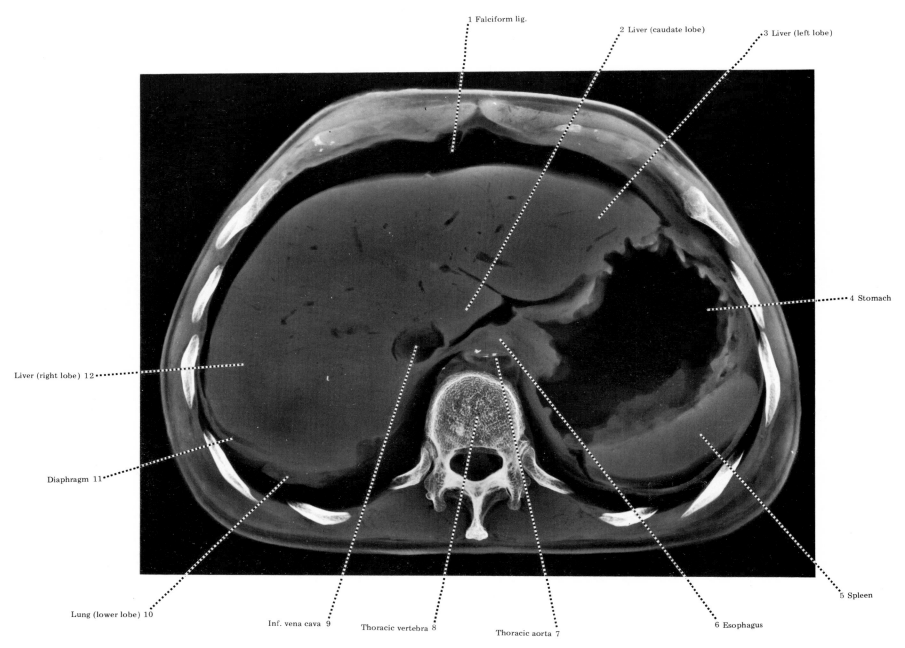

1 Falciform lig.

2 Liver (caudate lobe)

3 Liver (left lobe)

4 Stomach

Liver (right lobe) 12

Diaphragm 11

5 Spleen

Lung (lower lobe) 10

Inf. vena cava 9

Thoracic vertebra 8

Thoracic aorta 7

6 Esophagus

Section 27 (x-ray)

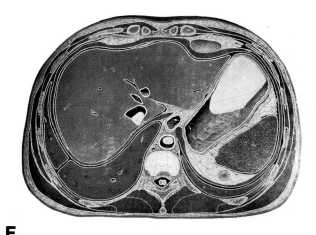

F

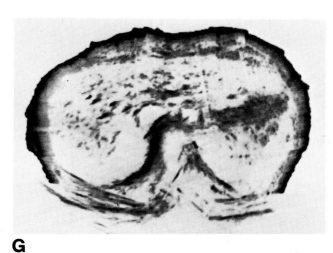

G

SECTION 27 (cont.)

Figure (**F**) is Section 27 reversed. In the echogram (**G**), the liver (2, 3, 12) presents as a fairly homogeneous structure, with some increasing echoes towards the center. At this level, the left lobe (3) is quite large. The aorta (7) is identified just to the left of the midline, and the inferior vena cava (9) and a hepatic vein are seen in a more anterior position. Portions of the spleen (5) are also demonstrated at this level. The posterior chest wall is still quite thin, and there is some loss of information due to the lowermost extensions of the lung (10).

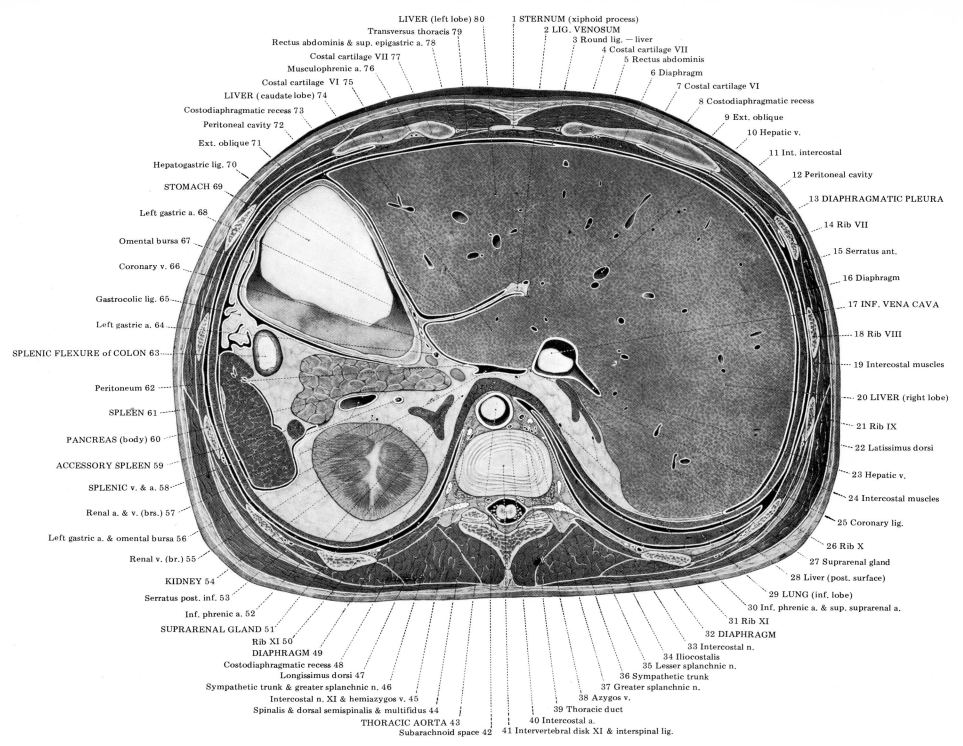

LIVER (left lobe) 80
Transversus thoracis 79
Rectus abdominis & sup. epigastric a. 78
Costal cartilage VII 77
Musculophrenic a. 76
Costal cartilage VI 75
LIVER (caudate lobe) 74
Costodiaphragmatic recess 73
Peritoneal cavity 72
Ext. oblique 71
Hepatogastric lig. 70
STOMACH 69
Left gastric a. 68
Omental bursa 67
Coronary v. 66
Gastrocolic lig. 65
Left gastric a. 64
SPLENIC FLEXURE of COLON 63
Peritoneum 62
SPLEEN 61
PANCREAS (body) 60
ACCESSORY SPLEEN 59
SPLENIC v. & a. 58
Renal a. & v. (brs.) 57
Left gastric a. & omental bursa 56
Renal v. (br.) 55
KIDNEY 54
Serratus post. inf. 53
Inf. phrenic a. 52
SUPRARENAL GLAND 51
Rib XI 50
DIAPHRAGM 49
Costodiaphragmatic recess 48
Longissimus dorsi 47
Sympathetic trunk & greater splanchnic n. 46
Intercostal n. XI & hemiazygos v. 45
Spinalis & dorsal semispinalis & multifidus 44
THORACIC AORTA 43
Subarachnoid space 42

1 STERNUM (xiphoid process)
2 LIG. VENOSUM
3 Round lig. — liver
4 Costal cartilage VII
5 Rectus abdominis
6 Diaphragm
7 Costal cartilage VI
8 Costodiaphragmatic recess
9 Ext. oblique
10 Hepatic v.
11 Int. intercostal
12 Peritoneal cavity
13 DIAPHRAGMATIC PLEURA
14 Rib VII
15 Serratus ant.
16 Diaphragm
17 INF. VENA CAVA
18 Rib VIII
19 Intercostal muscles
20 LIVER (right lobe)
21 Rib IX
22 Latissimus dorsi
23 Hepatic v.
24 Intercostal muscles
25 Coronary lig.
26 Rib X
27 Suprarenal gland
28 Liver (post. surface)
29 LUNG (inf. lobe)
30 Inf. phrenic a. & sup. suprarenal a.
31 Rib XI
32 DIAPHRAGM
33 Intercostal n.
34 Iliocostalis
35 Lesser splanchnic n.
36 Sympathetic trunk
37 Greater splanchnic n.
38 Azygos v.
39 Thoracic duct
40 Intercostal a.
41 Intervertebral disk XI & interspinal lig.

Section 28

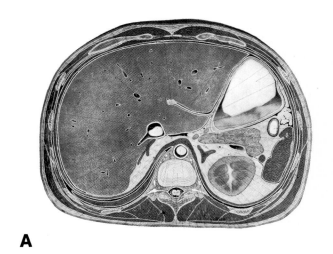

A

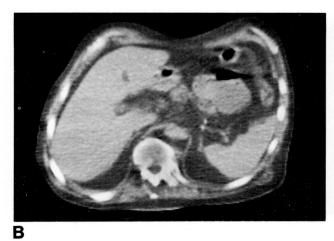

B

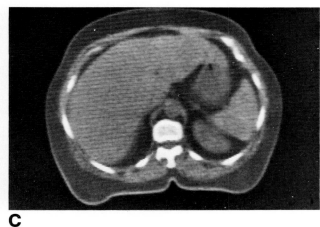

C

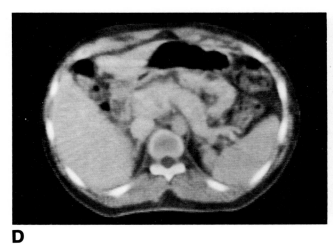

D

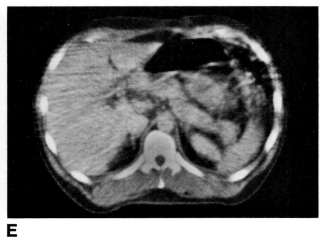

E

SECTION 28

Figure (**A**) is Section 28 reversed. The caudate lobe of the liver (**B, E**-74) lies adjacent to the vena cava (17) and is visible, as are the right (20) and left (80) lobes of the liver. The region of the main hepatic ducts can also be seen (**B, E**). The body and tail of the pancreas are usually identified (**D**-60, **E**-60) at the same level as the hilus of the spleen (61). Splenic vessels (58) and stomach (69) may blend in with the body and tail of the pancreas whereas the duodenum is close to the head of the pancreas. Note that the aorta (43) is enclosed by the diaphragm (32) and the superior mesenteric artery lies anterior to the aorta. The flat right adrenal gland (**D**-27, **E**-27) lies posterior to the vena cava (17), whereas the left adrenal gland (**D, E**-51) lies anteromedial to the upper pole of the left kidney (**E**-54).

Section 28

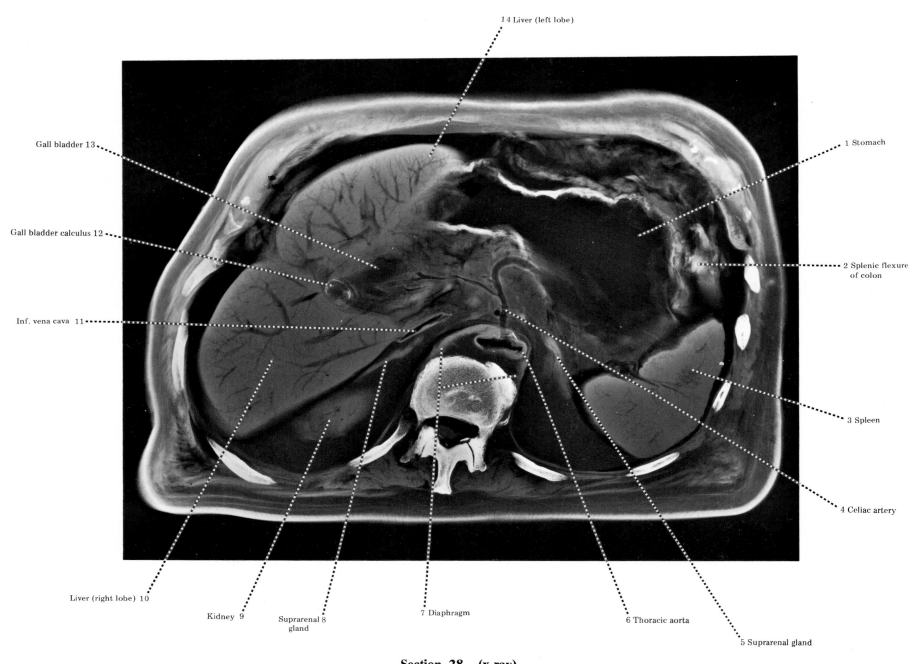

14 Liver (left lobe)

Gall bladder 13

Gall bladder calculus 12

Inf. vena cava 11

1 Stomach

2 Splenic flexure
of colon

3 Spleen

4 Celiac artery

Liver (right lobe) 10

Kidney 9

Suprarenal 8
gland

7 Diaphragm

6 Thoracic aorta

5 Suprarenal gland

Section 28 (x-ray)

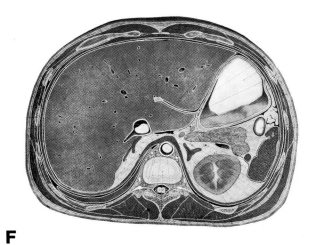

F

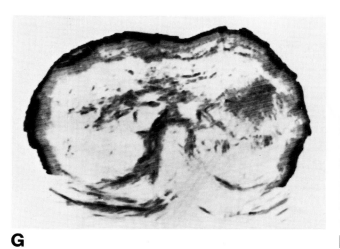

G

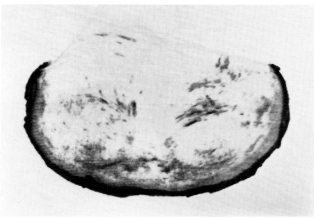

H

SECTION 28 (cont.)

Figure (**F**) is Section 28 reversed. In the echogram (anterior view, **G**), the left lobe of the liver (14) now appears as a thinner structure, and the upper pole of the kidney (9) is identified to the left of the spine. The spleen (3) is seen posterolateral to the kidney and the structure just anterolateral is a portion of the tail of the pancreas. The hilar echoes of the liver stand out particularly well on this section. The posterior view (**H**) at this level is limited because of the ribs and lung.

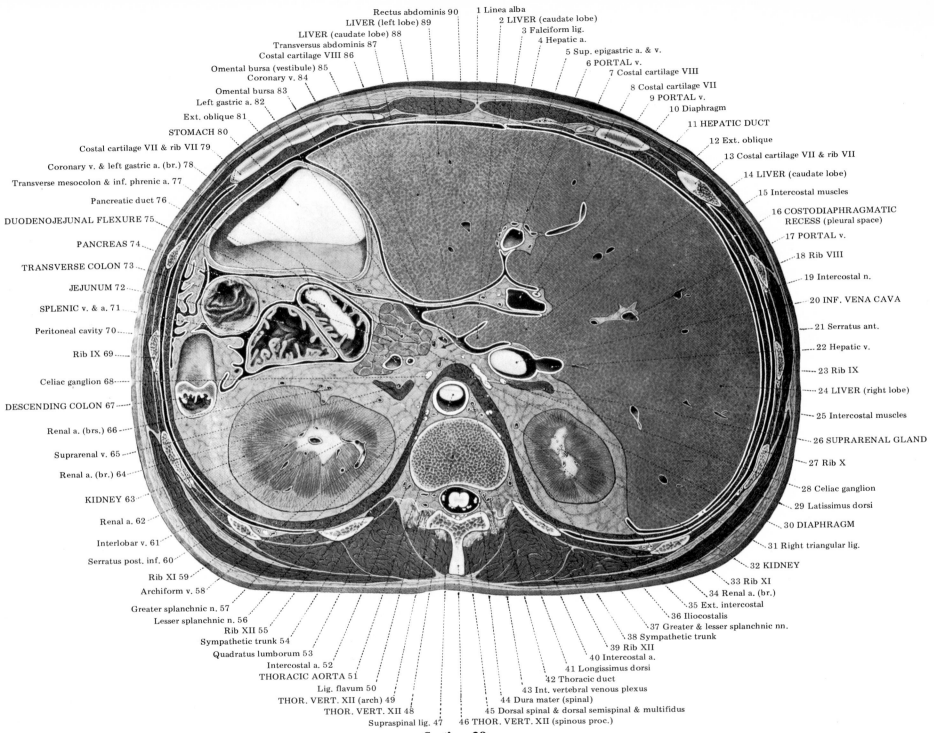

Rectus abdominis 90
LIVER (left lobe) 89
LIVER (caudate lobe) 88
Transversus abdominis 87
Costal cartilage VIII 86
Omental bursa (vestibule) 85
Coronary v. 84
Omental bursa 83
Left gastric a. 82
Ext. oblique 81
STOMACH 80
Costal cartilage VII & rib VII 79
Coronary v. & left gastric a. (br.) 78
Transverse mesocolon & inf. phrenic a. 77
Pancreatic duct 76
DUODENOJEJUNAL FLEXURE 75
PANCREAS 74
TRANSVERSE COLON 73
JEJUNUM 72
SPLENIC v. & a. 71
Peritoneal cavity 70
Rib IX 69
Celiac ganglion 68
DESCENDING COLON 67
Renal a. (brs.) 66
Suprarenal v. 65
Renal a. (br.) 64
KIDNEY 63
Renal a. 62
Interlobar v. 61
Serratus post. inf. 60
Rib XI 59
Archiform v. 58
Greater splanchnic n. 57
Lesser splanchnic n. 56
Rib XII 55
Sympathetic trunk 54
Quadratus lumborum 53
Intercostal a. 52
THORACIC AORTA 51
Lig. flavum 50
THOR. VERT. XII (arch) 49
THOR. VERT. XII 48
Supraspinal lig. 47

1 Linea alba
2 LIVER (caudate lobe)
3 Falciform lig.
4 Hepatic a.
5 Sup. epigastric a. & v.
6 PORTAL v.
7 Costal cartilage VIII
8 Costal cartilage VII
9 PORTAL v.
10 Diaphragm
11 HEPATIC DUCT
12 Ext. oblique
13 Costal cartilage VII & rib VII
14 LIVER (caudate lobe)
15 Intercostal muscles
16 COSTODIAPHRAGMATIC
RECESS (pleural space)
17 PORTAL v.
18 Rib VIII
19 Intercostal n.
20 INF. VENA CAVA
21 Serratus ant.
22 Hepatic v.
23 Rib IX
24 LIVER (right lobe)
25 Intercostal muscles
26 SUPRARENAL GLAND
27 Rib X
28 Celiac ganglion
29 Latissimus dorsi
30 DIAPHRAGM
31 Right triangular lig.
32 KIDNEY
33 Rib XI
34 Renal a. (br.)
35 Ext. intercostal
36 Iliocostalis
37 Greater & lesser splanchnic nn.
38 Sympathetic trunk
39 Rib XII
40 Intercostal a.
41 Longissimus dorsi
42 Thoracic duct
43 Int. vertebral venous plexus
44 Dura mater (spinal)
45 Dorsal spinal & dorsal semispinal & multifidus
46 THOR. VERT. XII (spinous proc.)

Section 29

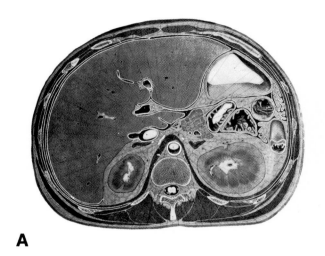

A

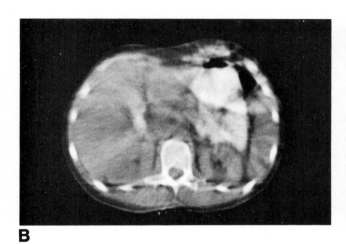

B

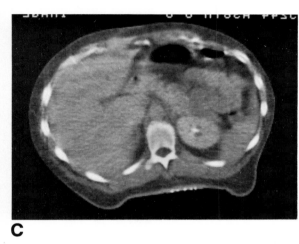

C

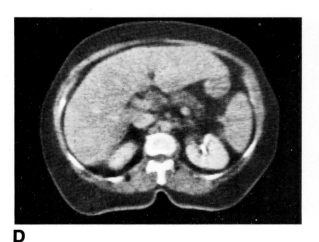

D

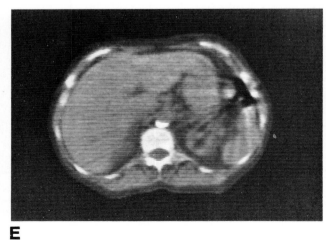

E

SECTION 29

Figure (**A**) is Section 29 reversed. The vena cava (20) lies posteromedial to the caudate lobe of the liver (2) and is faintly opacified (**D**) to the right of the aorta (51) which is enclosed by the diaphragm (30). The right kidney (32) lies medial to the right lobe of the liver (24), whereas the left kidney (63) is seen in close proximity to the jejunum (**B**-72) and pancreas (**C**-74). The splenic vein (**D**-71) is faintly opacified and can be seen behind the pancreas. The portal vein (**D**-9) which is barely opacified lies immediately anterior to the caudate lobe of the liver, and its branches can be faintly seen within the liver (**D**-17). Intravenous contrast material was used in Figures (**C**) and (**D**), and dilute Gastrografin * was used in (**B**). Jejunal loops (**B**-72) can be seen within the left side of the abdomen and the duodenum lies on the right. The stomach (80) is seen anteriorly and the spleen is evident laterally.

* Meglumine diatrizoate (66%) and sodium diatrizoate (10%) oral solution, E. R. Squibb & Sons

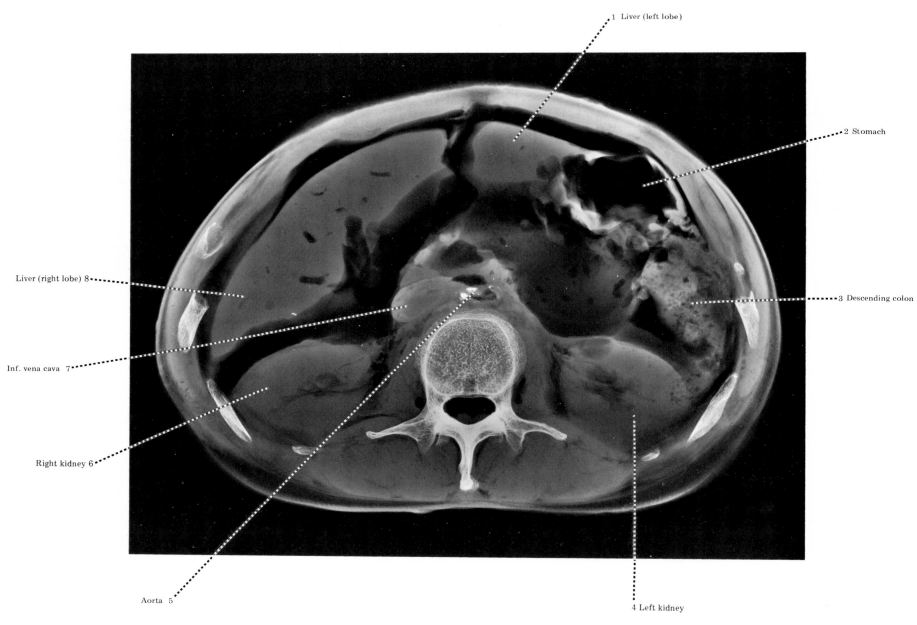

1 Liver (left lobe)

2 Stomach

3 Descending colon

Liver (right lobe) 8

Inf. vena cava 7

Right kidney 6

Aorta 5

4 Left kidney

Section 29 (x-ray)

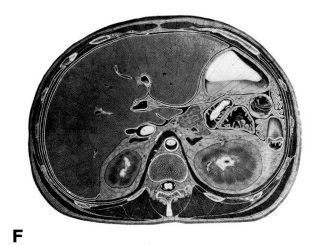

F

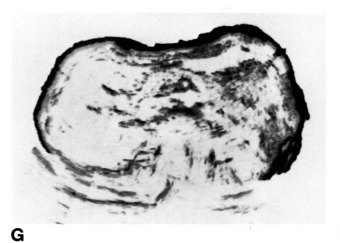

G

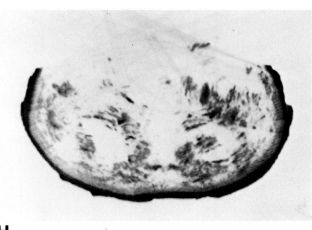

H

SECTION 29 (cont.)

Figure (**F**) is Section 29 reversed. In the echogram (anterior view, **G**), the right lobe (8) and hilar structures of the liver are seen. The upper portion of the superior mesenteric artery can be seen almost in the middle anterior to the aorta (5). Anterior to this, the body of the pancreas is seen. The echo-free area anteriorly and to the left represents fluid-filled stomach. Bowel loops obscure the visualization of the remainder of the left side of the abdomen. Posteriorly (**H**), the kidneys (4) are both well displayed.

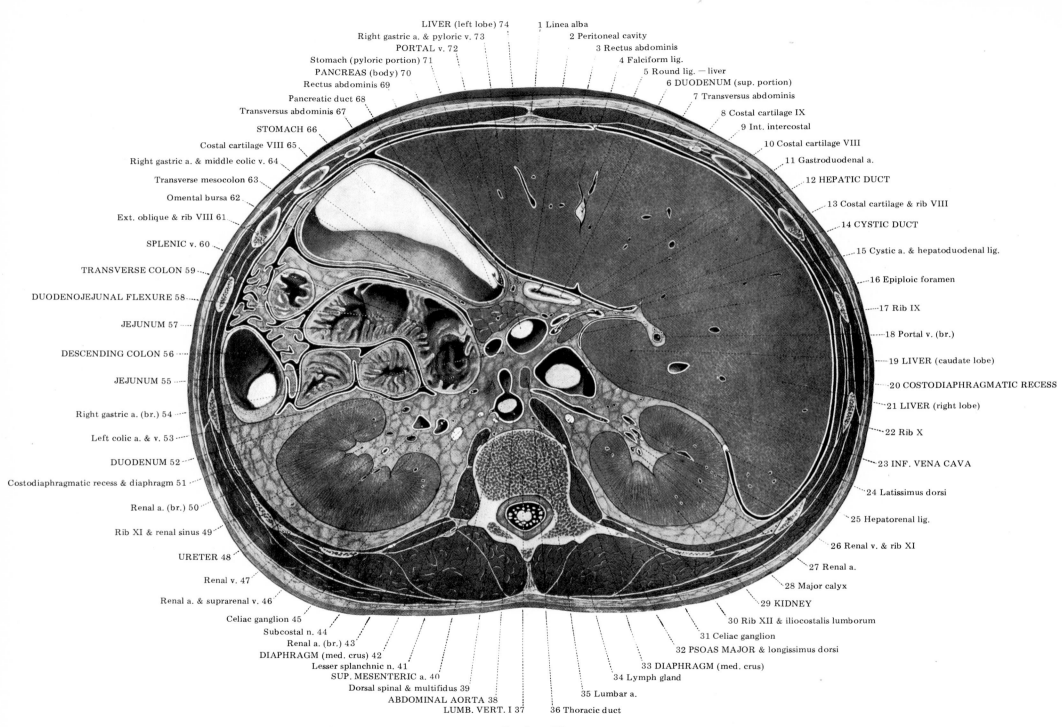

LIVER (left lobe) 74
Right gastric a. & pyloric v. 73
PORTAL v. 72
Stomach (pyloric portion) 71
PANCREAS (body) 70
Rectus abdominis 69
Pancreatic duct 68
Transversus abdominis 67
STOMACH 66
Costal cartilage VIII 65
Right gastric a. & middle colic v. 64
Transverse mesocolon 63
Omental bursa 62
Ext. oblique & rib VIII 61
SPLENIC v. 60
TRANSVERSE COLON 59
DUODENOJEJUNAL FLEXURE 58
JEJUNUM 57
DESCENDING COLON 56
JEJUNUM 55
Right gastric a. (br.) 54
Left colic a. & v. 53
DUODENUM 52
Costodiaphragmatic recess & diaphragm 51
Renal a. (br.) 50
Rib XI & renal sinus 49
URETER 48
Renal v. 47
Renal a. & suprarenal v. 46
Celiac ganglion 45
Subcostal n. 44
Renal a. (br.) 43
DIAPHRAGM (med. crus) 42
Lesser splanchnic n. 41
SUP. MESENTERIC a. 40
Dorsal spinal & multifidus 39
ABDOMINAL AORTA 38
LUMB. VERT. I 37

1 Linea alba
2 Peritoneal cavity
3 Rectus abdominis
4 Falciform lig.
5 Round lig. — liver
6 DUODENUM (sup. portion)
7 Transversus abdominis
8 Costal cartilage IX
9 Int. intercostal
10 Costal cartilage VIII
11 Gastroduodenal a.
12 HEPATIC DUCT
13 Costal cartilage & rib VIII
14 CYSTIC DUCT
15 Cystic a. & hepatoduodenal lig.
16 Epiploic foramen
17 Rib IX
18 Portal v. (br.)
19 LIVER (caudate lobe)
20 COSTODIAPHRAGMATIC RECESS
21 LIVER (right lobe)
22 Rib X
23 INF. VENA CAVA
24 Latissimus dorsi
25 Hepatorenal lig.
26 Renal v. & rib XI
27 Renal a.
28 Major calyx
29 KIDNEY
30 Rib XII & iliocostalis lumborum
31 Celiac ganglion
32 PSOAS MAJOR & longissimus dorsi
33 DIAPHRAGM (med. crus)
34 Lymph gland
35 Lumbar a.
36 Thoracic duct

Section 30

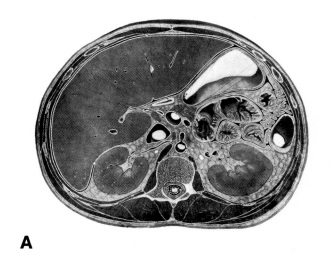

A

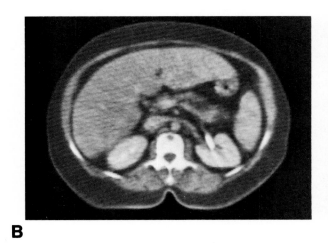

B

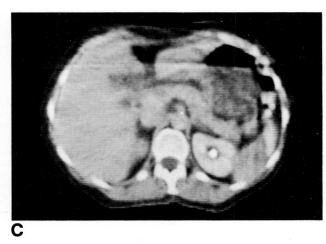

C

SECTION 30

Figure (**A**) is Section 30 reversed. The body of the pancreas (70) can usually be identified from the position of the superior mesenteric artery (**C**-40) where it originates from the aorta (38). However, the pancreas is in close proximity to and must be differentiated from other structures such as duodenum, stomach (**C**-66), jejunum, splenic and portal veins, as well as from inferior vena cava. Two or three scans may be required to encompass the whole pancreas because of its oblique position within the abdomen. Figures (**B**) and (**D**) show renal veins (26) draining into the vena cava (23) with the superior mesenteric artery (40) anterior to the renal vein (26), and the portal vein (72) anterior to the vena cava (23). Note how the vena cava simulates the head of the pancreas (**C**). The medial crus of the diaphragm (42) is adjacent to the spine (37) and aorta (38). Right (21) and left (74) lobes of the liver are seen as is the spleen, (**B**) and (**C**). The collecting systems are opacified within the kidneys (29) by intravenous contrast material. Stomach (66), jejunum (55), and colon (56) are anterior to the left kidney.

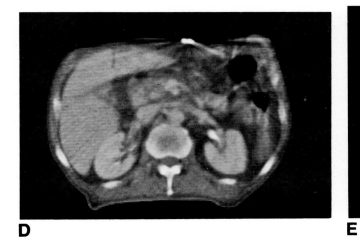

D

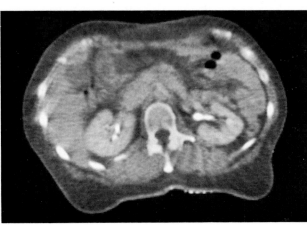

E

Section 30

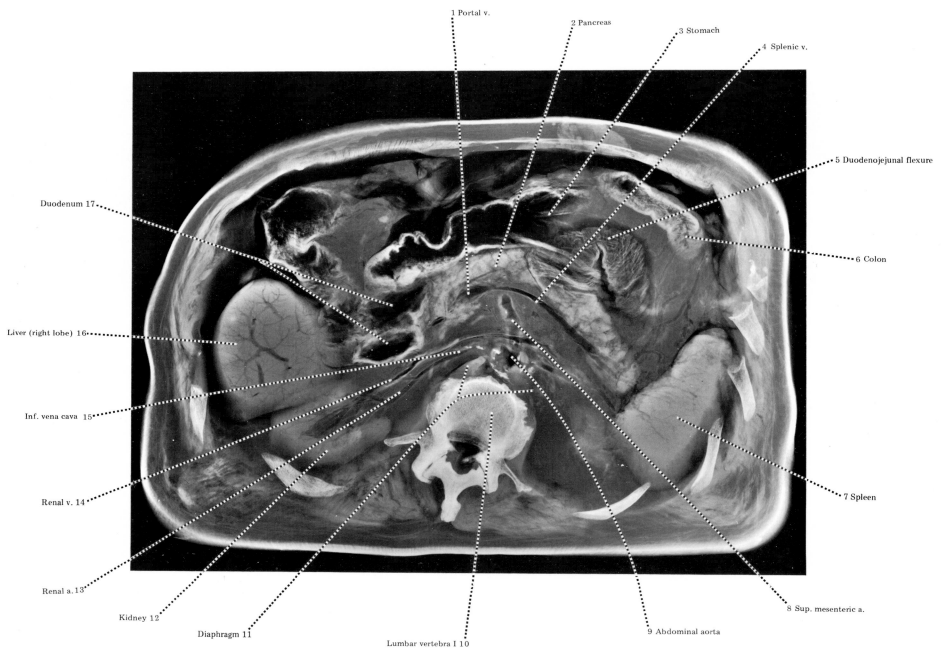

1 Portal v.

2 Pancreas

3 Stomach

4 Splenic v.

5 Duodenojejunal flexure

Duodenum 17

6 Colon

Liver (right lobe) 16

Inf. vena cava 15

7 Spleen

Renal v. 14

Renal a. 13

8 Sup. mesenteric a.

Kidney 12

9 Abdominal aorta

Diaphragm 11

Lumbar vertebra I 10

Section 30 (x-ray)

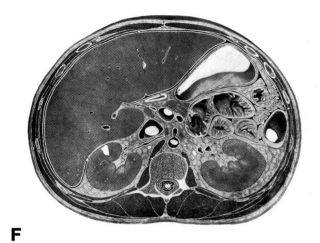

F

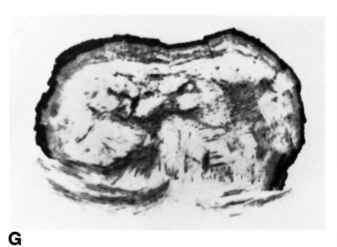

G

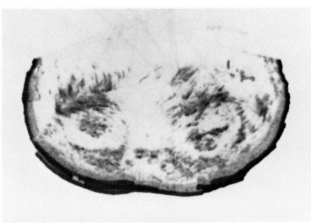

H

SECTION 30 (cont.)

Figure (**F**) is Section 30 reversed. In the echogram (anterior view, **G**), the superior mesenteric artery (8) is seen just anterior to the aorta (9), and the pancreas (2) is seen to the right. Note the relationship of the pancreas to the inferior vena cava (15). The right kidney is seen through the liver, but its margin is not sharply demarcated. The posterior view (**H**) gives excellent demonstration of both kidneys (12).

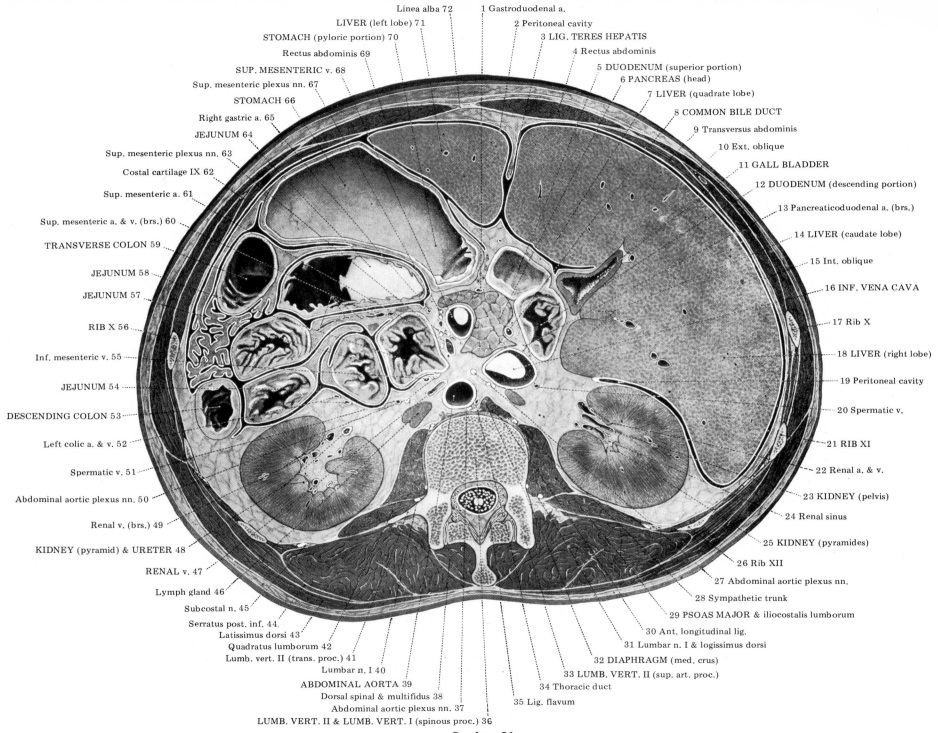

Linea alba 72
LIVER (left lobe) 71
STOMACH (pyloric portion) 70
Rectus abdominis 69
SUP. MESENTERIC v. 68
Sup. mesenteric plexus nn. 67
STOMACH 66
Right gastric a. 65
JEJUNUM 64
Sup. mesenteric plexus nn. 63
Costal cartilage IX 62
Sup. mesenteric a. 61
Sup. mesenteric a. & v. (brs.) 60
TRANSVERSE COLON 59
JEJUNUM 58
JEJUNUM 57
RIB X 56
Inf. mesenteric v. 55
JEJUNUM 54
DESCENDING COLON 53
Left colic a. & v. 52
Spermatic v. 51
Abdominal aortic plexus nn. 50
Renal v. (brs.) 49
KIDNEY (pyramid) & URETER 48
RENAL v. 47
Lymph gland 46
Subcostal n. 45
Serratus post. inf. 44
Latissimus dorsi 43
Quadratus lumborum 42
Lumb. vert. II (trans. proc.) 41
Lumbar n. I 40
ABDOMINAL AORTA 39
Dorsal spinal & multifidus 38
Abdominal aortic plexus nn. 37
LUMB. VERT. II & LUMB. VERT. I (spinous proc.) 36

1 Gastroduodenal a.
2 Peritoneal cavity
3 LIG. TERES HEPATIS
4 Rectus abdominis
5 DUODENUM (superior portion)
6 PANCREAS (head)
7 LIVER (quadrate lobe)
8 COMMON BILE DUCT
9 Transversus abdominis
10 Ext. oblique
11 GALL BLADDER
12 DUODENUM (descending portion)
13 Pancreaticoduodenal a. (brs.)
14 LIVER (caudate lobe)
15 Int. oblique
16 INF. VENA CAVA
17 Rib X
18 LIVER (right lobe)
19 Peritoneal cavity
20 Spermatic v.
21 RIB XI
22 Renal a. & v.
23 KIDNEY (pelvis)
24 Renal sinus
25 KIDNEY (pyramides)
26 Rib XII
27 Abdominal aortic plexus nn.
28 Sympathetic trunk
29 PSOAS MAJOR & iliocostalis lumborum
30 Ant. longitudinal lig.
31 Lumbar n. I & logissimus dorsi
32 DIAPHRAGM (med. crus)
33 LUMB. VERT. II (sup. art. proc.)
34 Thoracic duct
35 Lig. flavum

Section 31

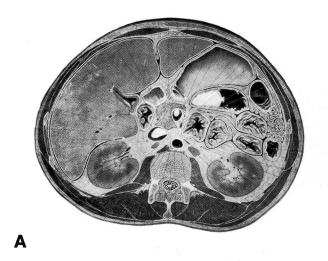

A

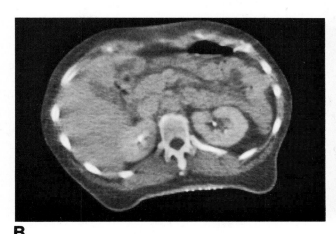

B

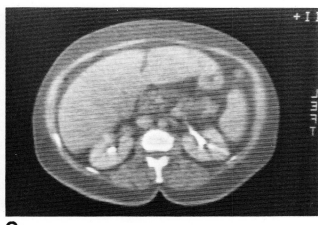

C

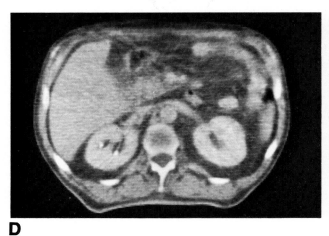

D

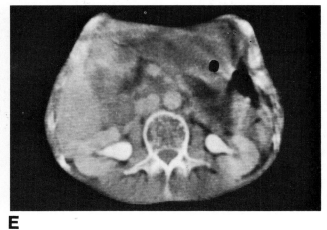

E

SECTION 31

Figure (**A**) is Section 31 reversed. The gallbladder (**B**-11) is usually seen along the inferior surface of the liver between the quadrate lobe (7) and caudate lobe (14). The ligamentum teres (3) separates the lateral segment of the left lobe (**C**-71) from the medial segment. The descending duodenum (12) is close to the liver (18) and the kidney (25), whereas the aorta (39) lies anterior to the spine (36). The vena cava (16) is posterior to the head of the pancreas (6) and is also close to the duodenum. The renal vein may be seen draining into the vena cava (16). Retroperitoneal nodes may be visible. Note that fat may surround the collecting system of the kidney and that an extra-renal pelvis may simulate a mass (**E**). Psoas muscles are also seen (**C, D, E**-29). All images were obtained following injection of intravenous contrast material.

Section 31

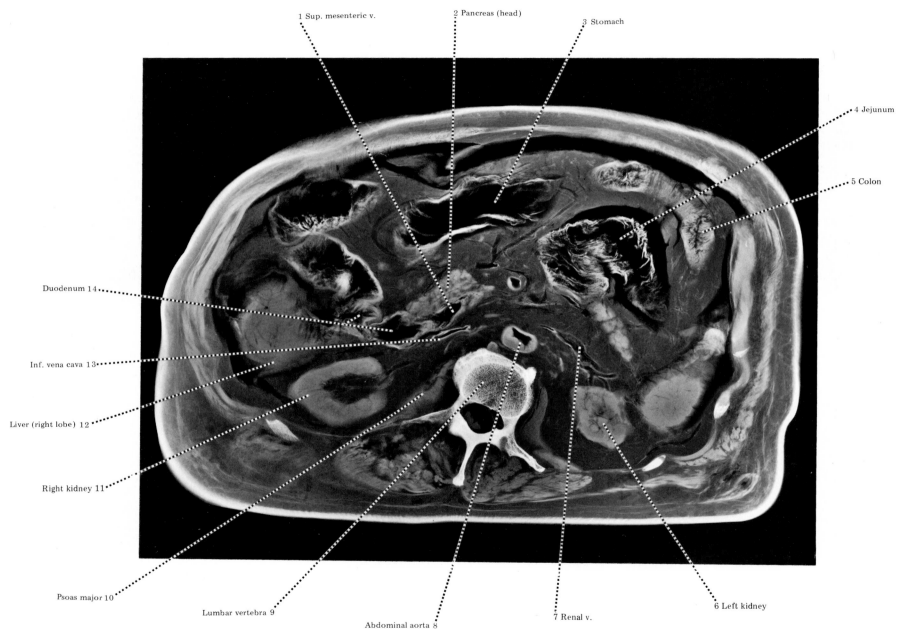

1 Sup. mesenteric v.

2 Pancreas (head)

3 Stomach

4 Jejunum

5 Colon

Duodenum 14

Inf. vena cava 13

Liver (right lobe) 12

Right kidney 11

Psoas major 10

Lumbar vertebra 9

Abdominal aorta 8

7 Renal v.

6 Left kidney

Section 31   (x-ray)

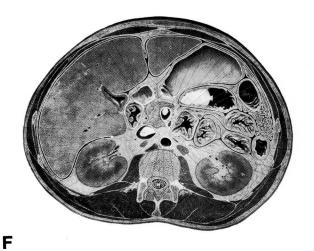

F

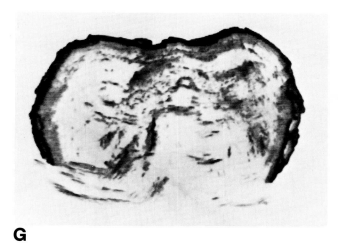

G

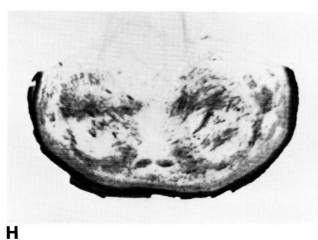

H

SECTION 31 (cont.)

Figure (**F**) is Section 31 reversed. In the echogram (anterior view, **G**), only a small portion of the right lobe of the liver (12) is visualized at this level. The kidney (11) is seen more clearly through the liver. The superior mesenteric artery is demonstrated anterior to the aorta (8), and a substantial portion of the pancreas (2) demonstrated anteriorly to the right. The left side of the abdomen is obscured by bowel echoes. Posteriorly (**H**), there is good demonstration of both kidneys (6, 11).

Section 31

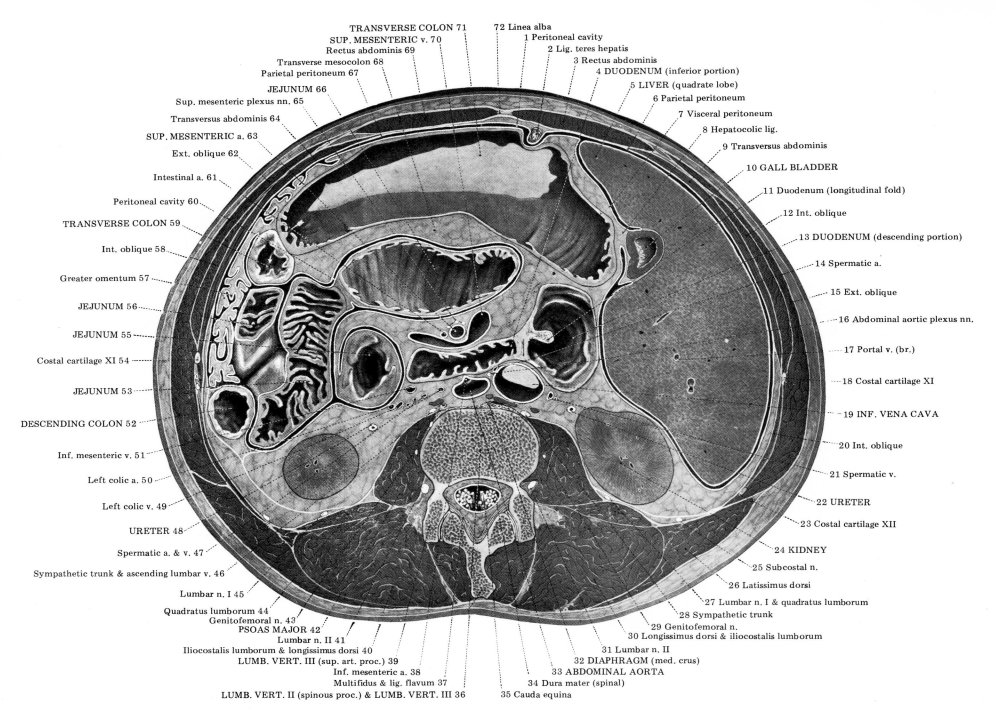

TRANSVERSE COLON 71
SUP. MESENTERIC v. 70
Rectus abdominis 69
Transverse mesocolon 68
Parietal peritoneum 67
JEJUNUM 66
Sup. mesenteric plexus nn. 65
Transversus abdominis 64
SUP. MESENTERIC a. 63
Ext. oblique 62
Intestinal a. 61
Peritoneal cavity 60
TRANSVERSE COLON 59
Int. oblique 58
Greater omentum 57
JEJUNUM 56
JEJUNUM 55
Costal cartilage XI 54
JEJUNUM 53
DESCENDING COLON 52
Inf. mesenteric v. 51
Left colic a. 50
Left colic v. 49
URETER 48
Spermatic a. & v. 47
Sympathetic trunk & ascending lumbar v. 46
Lumbar n. I 45
Quadratus lumborum 44
Genitofemoral n. 43
PSOAS MAJOR 42
Lumbar n. II 41
Iliocostalis lumborum & longissimus dorsi 40
LUMB. VERT. III (sup. art. proc.) 39
Inf. mesenteric a. 38
Multifidus & lig. flavum 37
LUMB. VERT. II (spinous proc.) & LUMB. VERT. III 36

72 Linea alba
1 Peritoneal cavity
2 Lig. teres hepatis
3 Rectus abdominis
4 DUODENUM (inferior portion)
5 LIVER (quadrate lobe)
6 Parietal peritoneum
7 Visceral peritoneum
8 Hepatocolic lig.
9 Transversus abdominis
10 GALL BLADDER
11 Duodenum (longitudinal fold)
12 Int. oblique
13 DUODENUM (descending portion)
14 Spermatic a.
15 Ext. oblique
16 Abdominal aortic plexus nn.
17 Portal v. (br.)
18 Costal cartilage XI
19 INF. VENA CAVA
20 Int. oblique
21 Spermatic v.
22 URETER
23 Costal cartilage XII
24 KIDNEY
25 Subcostal n.
26 Latissimus dorsi
27 Lumbar n. I & quadratus lumborum
28 Sympathetic trunk
29 Genitofemoral n.
30 Longissimus dorsi & iliocostalis lumborum
31 Lumbar n. II
32 DIAPHRAGM (med. crus)
33 ABDOMINAL AORTA
34 Dura mater (spinal)
35 Cauda equina

Section 32

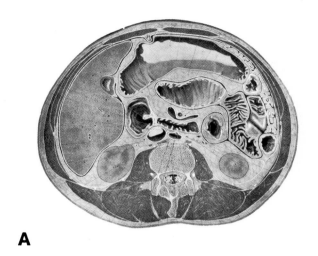

A

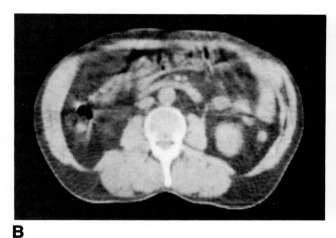

B

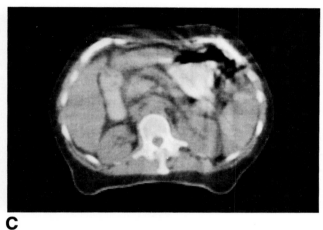

C

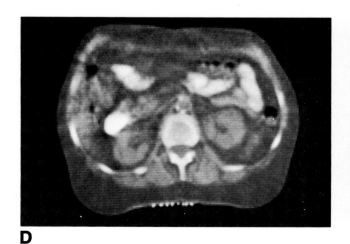

D

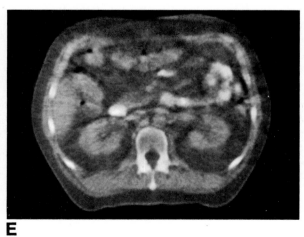

E

SECTION 32

Figure (**A**) is Section 32 reversed. The third portion of the duodenum (**B**-4) is retroperitoneal and passes immediately anterior to the aorta (33) and the vena cava (19). The superior mesenteric artery and vein (**B**-63, 70) are seen just anterior to the duodenum. The second portion of the duodenum (13) is anterior to the right kidney (24), whereas the jejunum (53) and colon (52) are anterior to the left kidney. Psoas muscles (42) are lateral to the vertebral body (36). There is considerable variation in the level of kidneys, liver, and spleen between various patients. Dilute Gastrografin * has been given to patients (**C, D, E**) to demonstrate relationships of bowel to the kidneys.

* Meglumine diatrizoate (66%) and sodium diatrizoate (10%) oral solution, E. R. Squibb & Sons

Section 32

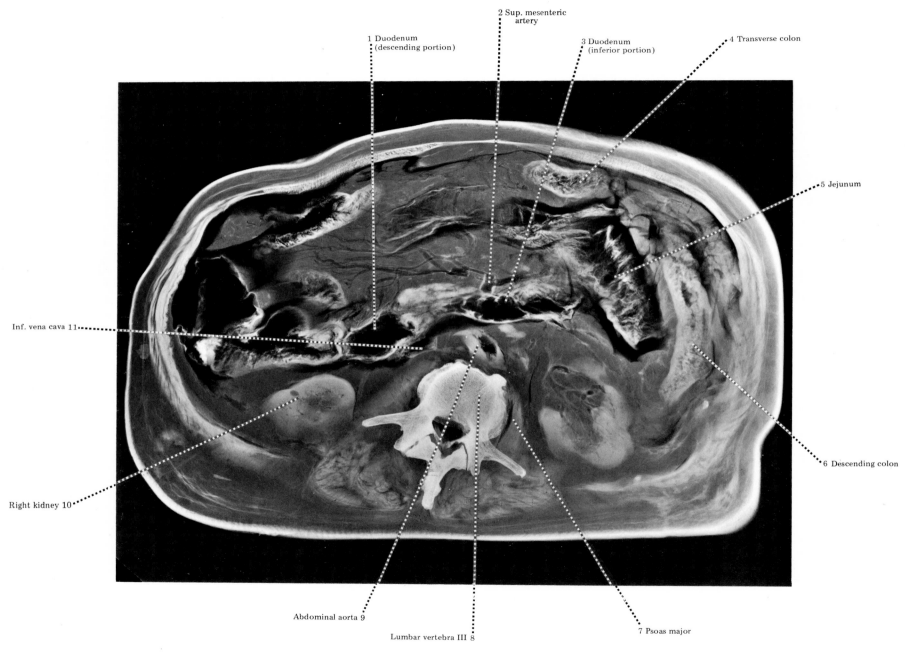

1 Duodenum (descending portion)

2 Sup. mesenteric artery

3 Duodenum (inferior portion)

4 Transverse colon

5 Jejunum

6 Descending colon

7 Psoas major

Inf. vena cava 11

Right kidney 10

Abdominal aorta 9

Lumbar vertebra III 8

Section 32 (x-ray)

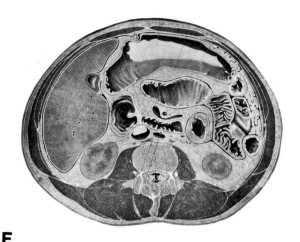

F

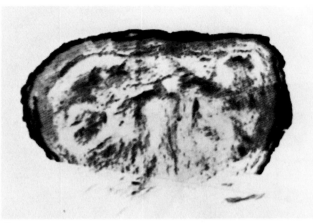

G

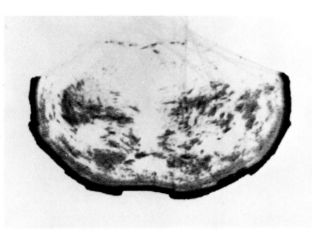

H

SECTION 32 (cont.)

Figure (**F**) is Section 32 reversed. In the echogram (anterior view, **G**), the flattening of the inferior vena cava (11) as compared to the rounded aorta (9) is demonstrated. Only a thin portion of the right lobe of the liver remains, but the kidney (10) stands out sharply on the right side. The structures on the left side are obscured by bowel gas. Posteriorly (**H**), the lower poles of the kidneys can be identified. The psoas muscles (7) are larger and seen between the spine and kidneys (10).

Section 32

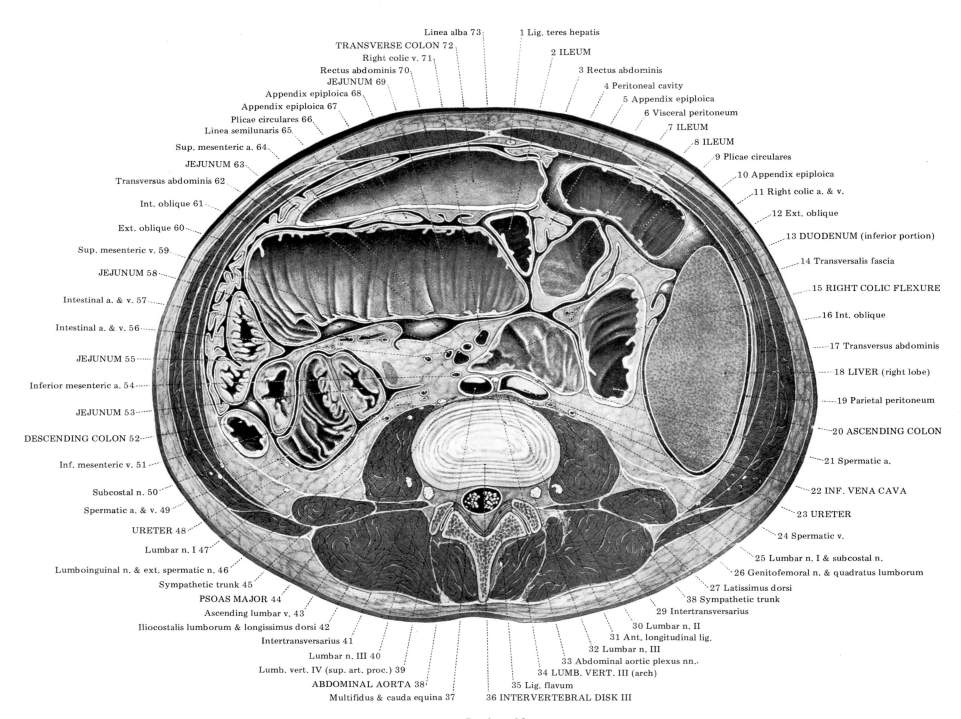

Linea alba 73
TRANSVERSE COLON 72
Right colic v. 71
Rectus abdominis 70
JEJUNUM 69
Appendix epiploica 68
Appendix epiploica 67
Plicae circulares 66
Linea semilunaris 65
Sup. mesenteric a. 64
JEJUNUM 63
Transversus abdominis 62
Int. oblique 61
Ext. oblique 60
Sup. mesenteric v. 59
JEJUNUM 58
Intestinal a. & v. 57
Intestinal a. & v. 56
JEJUNUM 55
Inferior mesenteric a. 54
JEJUNUM 53
DESCENDING COLON 52
Inf. mesenteric v. 51
Subcostal n. 50
Spermatic a. & v. 49
URETER 48
Lumbar n. I 47
Lumboinguinal n. & ext. spermatic n. 46
Sympathetic trunk 45
PSOAS MAJOR 44
Ascending lumbar v. 43
Iliocostalis lumborum & longissimus dorsi 42
Intertransversarius 41
Lumbar n. III 40
Lumb. vert. IV (sup. art. proc.) 39
ABDOMINAL AORTA 38
Multifidus & cauda equina 37

1 Lig. teres hepatis
2 ILEUM
3 Rectus abdominis
4 Peritoneal cavity
5 Appendix epiploica
6 Visceral peritoneum
7 ILEUM
8 ILEUM
9 Plicae circulares
10 Appendix epiploica
11 Right colic a. & v.
12 Ext. oblique
13 DUODENUM (inferior portion)
14 Transversalis fascia
15 RIGHT COLIC FLEXURE
16 Int. oblique
17 Transversus abdominis
18 LIVER (right lobe)
19 Parietal peritoneum
20 ASCENDING COLON
21 Spermatic a.
22 INF. VENA CAVA
23 URETER
24 Spermatic v.
25 Lumbar n. I & subcostal n.
26 Genitofemoral n. & quadratus lumborum
27 Latissimus dorsi
38 Sympathetic trunk
29 Intertransversarius
30 Lumbar n. II
31 Ant. longitudinal lig.
32 Lumbar n. III
33 Abdominal aortic plexus nn.
34 LUMB. VERT. III (arch)
35 Lig. flavum
36 INTERVERTEBRAL DISK III

Section 33

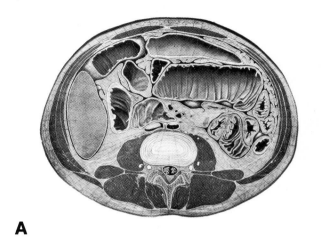

A

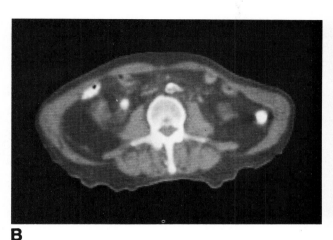

B

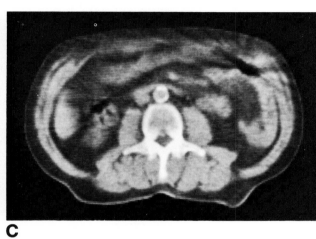

C

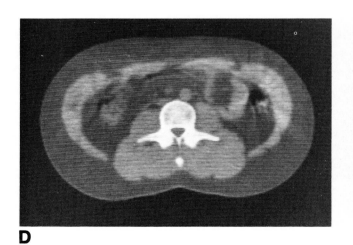

D

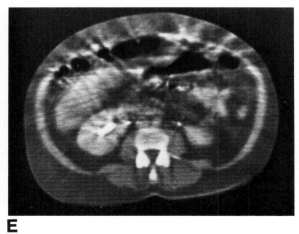

E

SECTION 33

Figure (**A**) is Section 33 reversed. The tip of the right lobe of the liver (**C**-18) may extend to below the lower pole of the kidneys. The aorta (38) is readily seen, particularly when its wall is calcified. The vena cava (22) is to the right of the aorta (38) and posterior to the third portion of the duodenum (**C**-13). The right (15) and left (52) colon are more easily identified when containing some contrast material (**B**). Note the variability of psoas muscles (44) and rectus abdominis (3, 70). Nonopacified ureters may occasionally be seen anterior to the psoas muscles (44) on plain CT scans (**C**) but are more easily seen when opacified (**E**-23, **E**-48).

Section 33

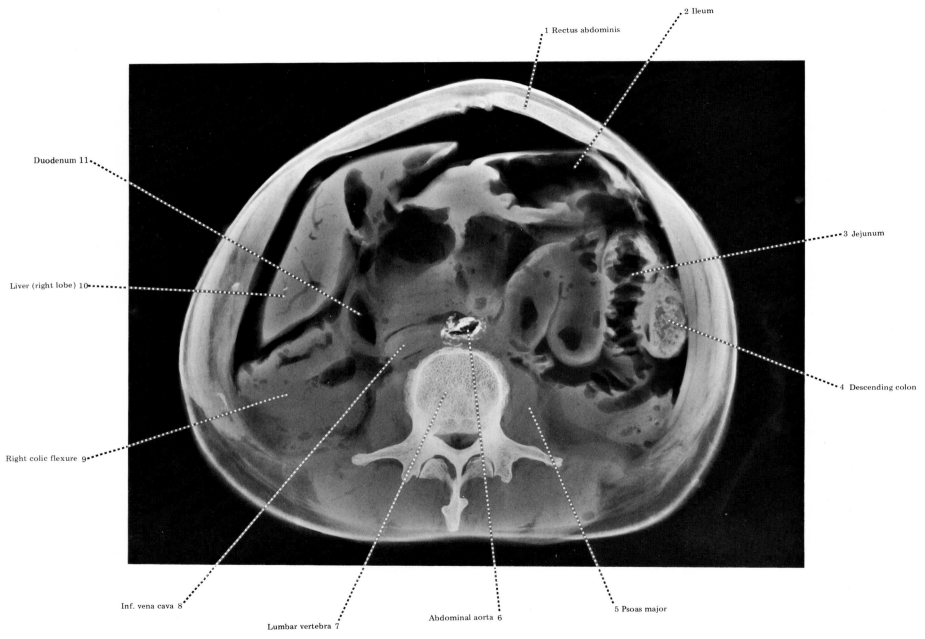

1 Rectus abdominis

2 Ileum

3 Jejunum

4 Descending colon

5 Psoas major

Abdominal aorta 6

Lumbar vertebra 7

Inf. vena cava 8

Right colic flexure 9

Liver (right lobe) 10

Duodenum 11

Section 33 (x-ray)

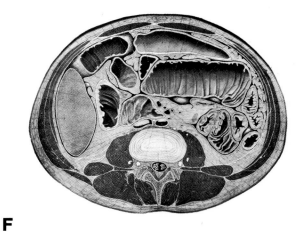

F

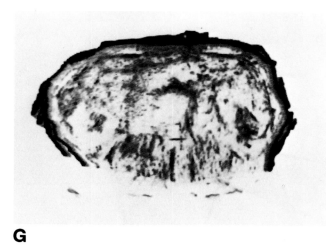

G

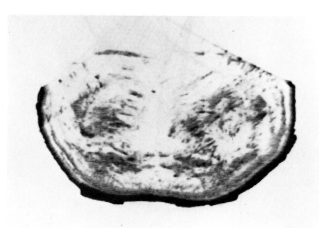

H

SECTION 33 (cont.)

Figure (**F**) is Section 33 reversed. In the echogram (anterior view, **G**), large amounts of gas preclude the visualization of all but the most anterior portions of the retroperitoneum, where the aorta (6) and inferior vena cava (8) are poorly defined. Most of the remaining abdominal echoes are produced by bowel structures. The lower pole of the right kidney can still be seen. Posteriorly (**H**), the increasing width of the back muscles is now apparent and the psoas muscles (5) can be seen just lateral to the shadow of the spine.

Section 33

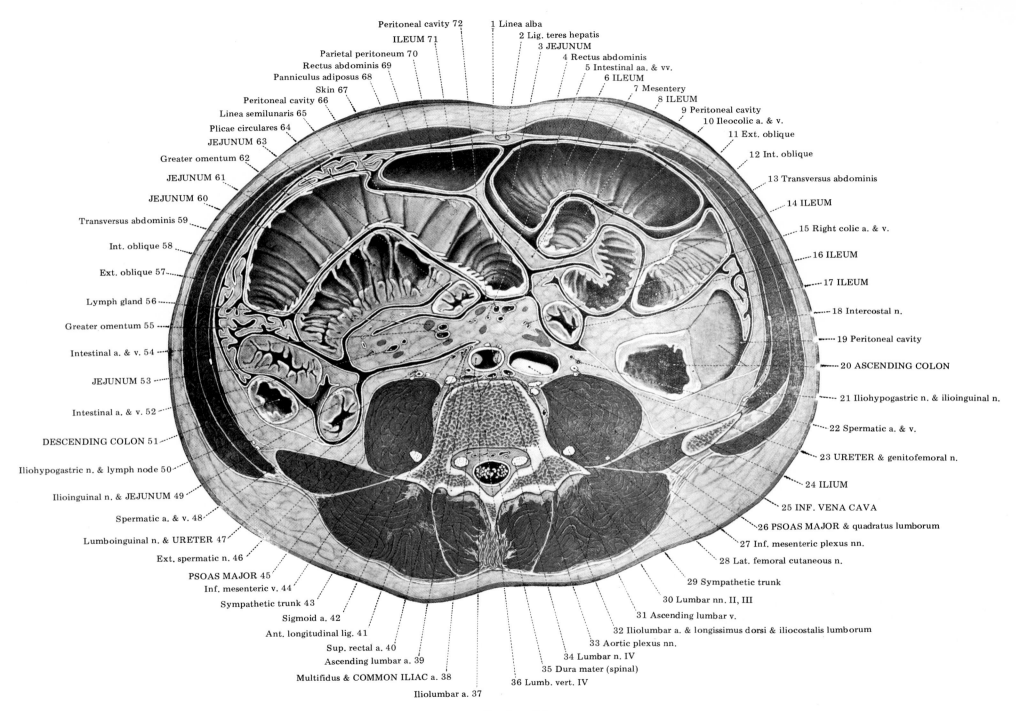

Peritoneal cavity 72
ILEUM 71
Parietal peritoneum 70
Rectus abdominis 69
Panniculus adiposus 68
Skin 67
Peritoneal cavity 66
Linea semilunaris 65
Plicae circulares 64
JEJUNUM 63
Greater omentum 62
JEJUNUM 61
JEJUNUM 60
Transversus abdominis 59
Int. oblique 58
Ext. oblique 57
Lymph gland 56
Greater omentum 55
Intestinal a. & v. 54
JEJUNUM 53
Intestinal a. & v. 52
DESCENDING COLON 51
Iliohypogastric n. & lymph node 50
Ilioinguinal n. & JEJUNUM 49
Spermatic a. & v. 48
Lumboinguinal n. & URETER 47
Ext. spermatic n. 46
PSOAS MAJOR 45
Inf. mesenteric v. 44
Sympathetic trunk 43
Sigmoid a. 42
Ant. longitudinal lig. 41
Sup. rectal a. 40
Ascending lumbar 39
Multifidus & COMMON ILIAC a. 38
Iliolumbar a. 37

1 Linea alba
2 Lig. teres hepatis
3 JEJUNUM
4 Rectus abdominis
5 Intestinal aa. & vv.
6 ILEUM
7 Mesentery
8 ILEUM
9 Peritoneal cavity
10 Ileocolic a. & v.
11 Ext. oblique
12 Int. oblique
13 Transversus abdominis
14 ILEUM
15 Right colic a. & v.
16 ILEUM
17 ILEUM
18 Intercostal n.
19 Peritoneal cavity
20 ASCENDING COLON
21 Iliohypogastric n. & ilioinguinal n.
22 Spermatic a. & v.
23 URETER & genitofemoral n.
24 ILIUM
25 INF. VENA CAVA
26 PSOAS MAJOR & quadratus lumborum
27 Inf. mesenteric plexus nn.
28 Lat. femoral cutaneous n.
29 Sympathetic trunk
30 Lumbar nn. II, III
31 Ascending lumbar v.
32 Iliolumbar a. & longissimus dorsi & iliocostalis lumborum
33 Aortic plexus nn.
34 Lumbar n. IV
35 Dura mater (spinal)
36 Lumb. vert. IV

Section 34

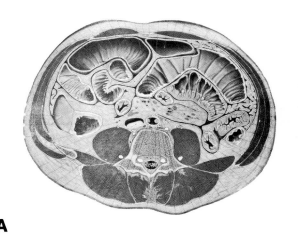

A

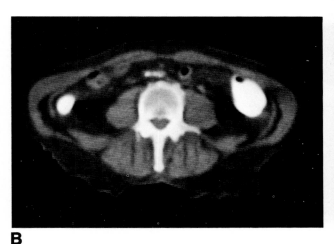

B

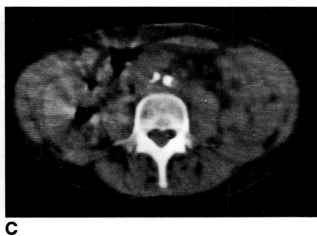

C

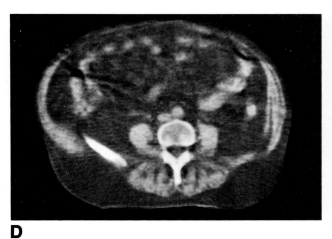

D

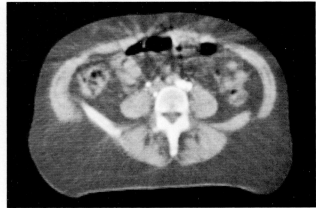

E

SECTION 34

Figure (**A**) is Section 34 reversed. These scans, taken at the level of iliac crest (**D**-24, **E**-24), are in the vicinity of the aortic bifurcation. The common iliac arteries are more easily identified when calcified (**B**-38, **C**-38). The colon is recognizable when containing contrast material (**B**-20, **B**-51). The vena cava (**D**-25) is seen to right of the aorta (**D**-38). Lymph nodes are opacified (**E**-50) following a lymphangiogram. Note how bowel loops tend to "float" in an obese patient (**D**). The psoas muscles (26) are lateral to the vertebral body (36), and various muscles of the abdominal wall can be seen: transverse (**D**-13), internal oblique (**D**-12), external oblique (**D**-11) can be separately identified.

Section 34

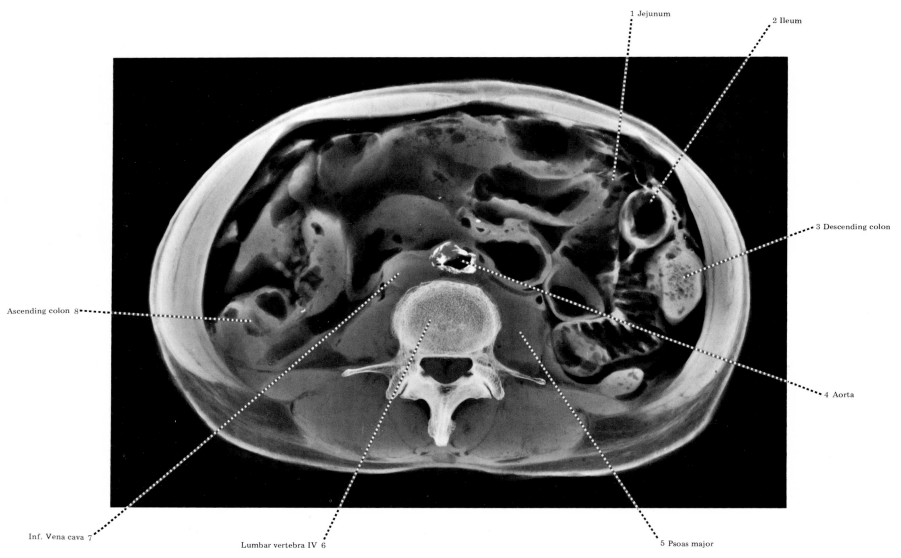

1 Jejunum

2 Ileum

3 Descending colon

4 Aorta

Ascending colon 8

Inf. Vena cava 7

Lumbar vertebra IV 6

5 Psoas major

Section 34   (x-ray)

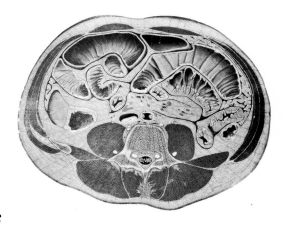

F

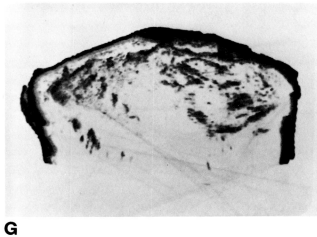

G

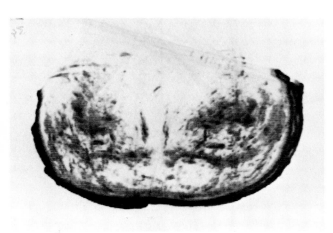

H

SECTION 34 (cont.)

Figure (**F**) is Section 34 reversed. In the echogram (anterior view, **G**), only the thin layer of abdominal wall muscles and peritoneum form anatomic landmarks at this level. Bowel loops containing considerable gas obscure the entire remainder of the abdomen from another view. Posteriorly (**H**), the mass of the longissimus dorsi is easily discernible. The increasing bulk of the psoas muscles (5) can be seen protruding lateral to the spine (6).

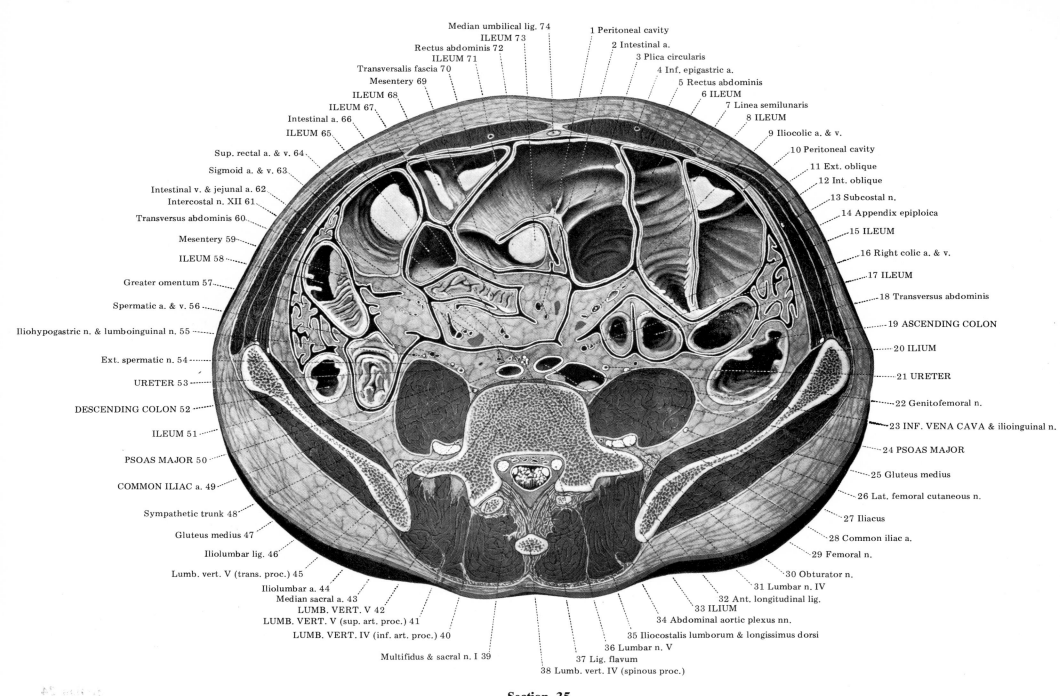

Median umbilical lig. 74
ILEUM 73
Rectus abdominis 72
ILEUM 71
Transversalis fascia 70
Mesentery 69
ILEUM 68
ILEUM 67
Intestinal a. 66
ILEUM 65
Sup. rectal a. & v. 64
Sigmoid a. & v. 63
Intestinal v. & jejunal a. 62
Intercostal n. XII 61
Transversus abdominis 60
Mesentery 59
ILEUM 58
Greater omentum 57
Spermatic a. & v. 56
Iliohypogastric n. & lumboinguinal n. 55
Ext. spermatic n. 54
URETER 53
DESCENDING COLON 52
ILEUM 51
PSOAS MAJOR 50
COMMON ILIAC a. 49
Sympathetic trunk 48
Gluteus medius 47
Iliolumbar lig. 46
Lumb. vert. V (trans. proc.) 45
Iliolumbar a. 44
Median sacral a. 43
LUMB. VERT. V 42
LUMB. VERT. V (sup. art. proc.) 41
LUMB. VERT. IV (inf. art. proc.) 40
Multifidus & sacral n. I 39

1 Peritoneal cavity
2 Intestinal a.
3 Plica circularis
4 Inf. epigastric a.
5 Rectus abdominis
6 ILEUM
7 Linea semilunaris
8 ILEUM
9 Iliocolic a. & v.
10 Peritoneal cavity
11 Ext. oblique
12 Int. oblique
13 Subcostal n.
14 Appendix epiploica
15 ILEUM
16 Right colic a. & v.
17 ILEUM
18 Transversus abdominis
19 ASCENDING COLON
20 ILIUM
21 URETER
22 Genitofemoral n.
23 INF. VENA CAVA & ilioinguinal n.
24 PSOAS MAJOR
25 Gluteus medius
26 Lat. femoral cutaneous n.
27 Iliacus
28 Common iliac a.
29 Femoral n.
30 Obturator n.
31 Lumbar n. IV
32 Ant. longitudinal lig.
33 ILIUM
34 Abdominal aortic plexus nn.
35 Iliocostalis lumborum & longissimus dorsi
36 Lumbar n. V
37 Lig. flavum
38 Lumb. vert. IV (spinous proc.)

Section 35

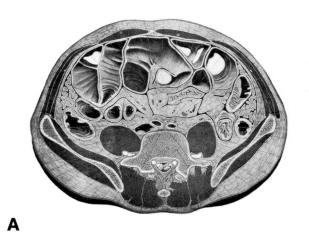

A

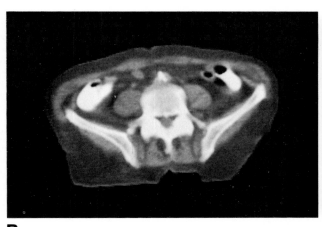

B

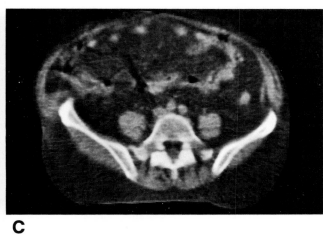

C

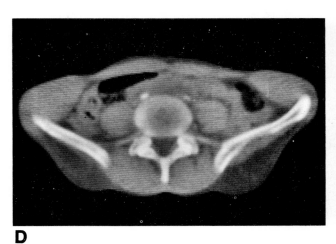

D

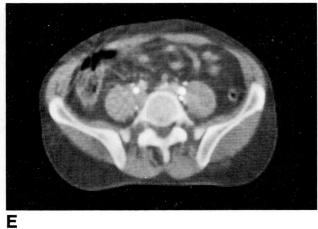

E

SECTION 35

Figure (**A**) is Section 35 reversed. At the level of L5 (42), the iliac bone (20) with iliac muscle (27) and gluteus medius (25) are clearly seen. Colon (**B**-19, **B**-52) is identified when containing contrast material. Small bowel loops containing fluid may tend to "float" on the mesenteric fat (**C**). The ureters (21, 53) lying anterior to psoas (24) are nonopacified (**B**). Lymph nodes may also be seen around psoas muscle (24) but are more readily identified when containing contrast material (**E**). Common iliac arteries (28, 49) are visible, particularly when calcified (**B, D**). The vena cava (**C**-23) is seen to the right of iliac arteries.

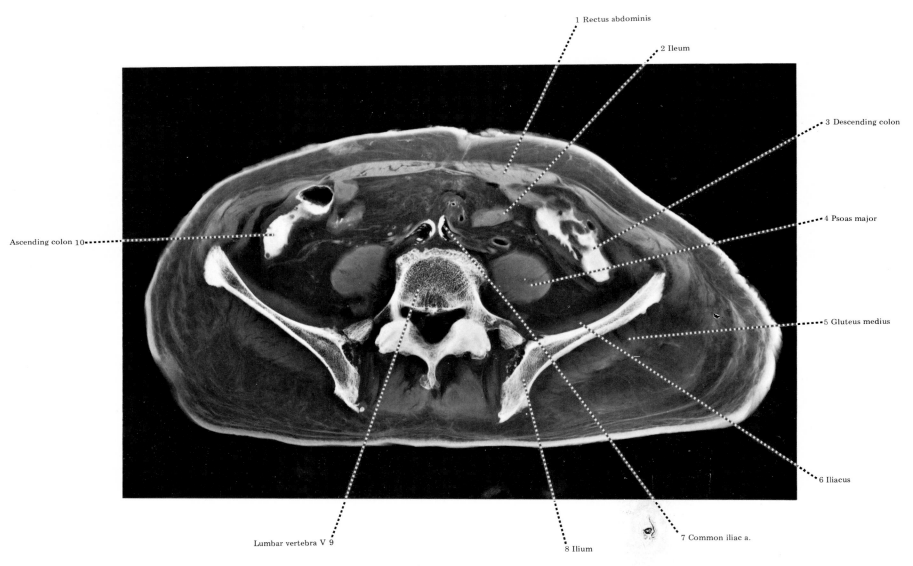

1 Rectus abdominis

2 Ileum

3 Descending colon

4 Psoas major

5 Gluteus medius

6 Iliacus

Ascending colon 10

Lumbar vertebra V 9

8 Ilium

7 Common iliac a.

Section 35 (x-ray)

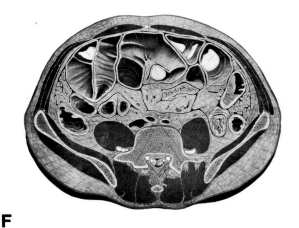

F

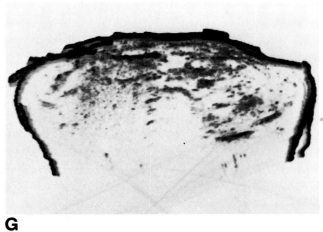

G

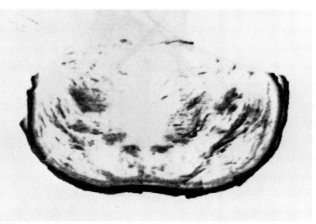

H

SECTION 35 (cont.)

Figure (**F**) is Section 35 reversed. In the echogram (anterior view, **G**), the rectus abdominis muscles (1) can be defined anteriorly but gas obscures most of the abdomen anteriorly. Laterally, the iliac crest can be defined, with some reflections of echoes from its medial surface. Posteriorly (**H**), the gluteus medius (5) is seen. The wide lumbar vertebral body (9) and iliac bone (8) prevent visualization of the psoas or anterior structures below this level. Thus, the posterior sections will no longer be included.

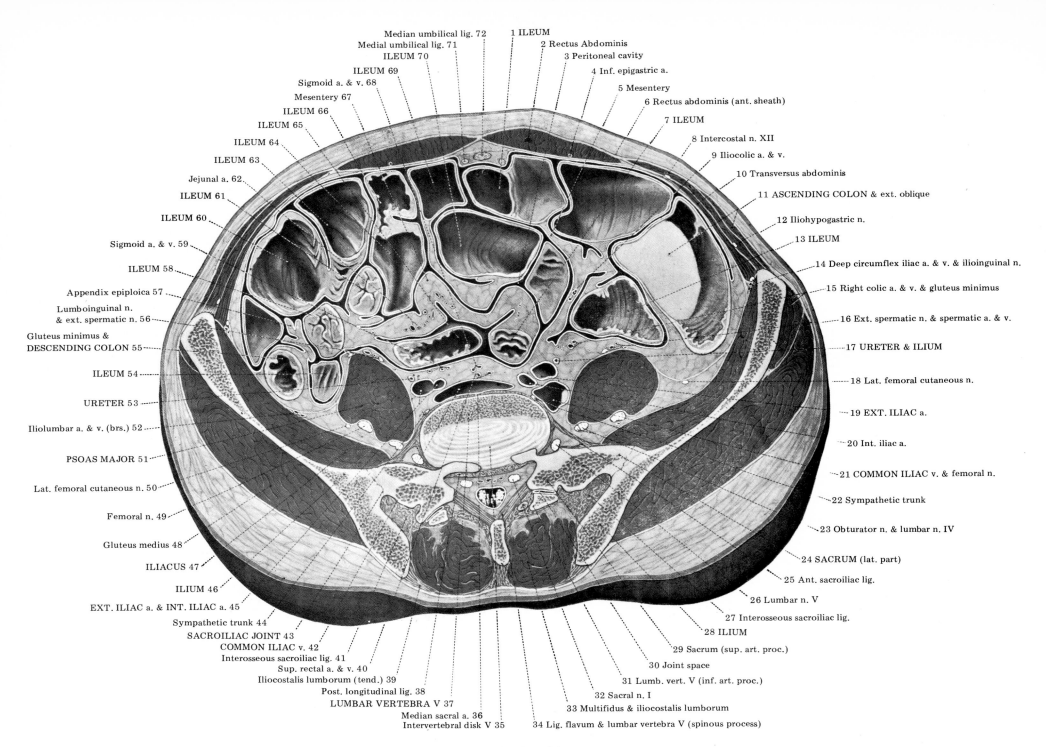

Median umbilical lig. 72
Medial umbilical lig. 71
ILEUM 70
ILEUM 69
Sigmoid a. & v. 68
Mesentery 67
ILEUM 66
ILEUM 65
ILEUM 64
ILEUM 63
Jejunal a. 62
ILEUM 61
ILEUM 60
Sigmoid a. & v. 59
ILEUM 58
Appendix epiploica 57
Lumboinguinal n.
& ext. spermatic n. 56
Gluteus minimus &
DESCENDING COLON 55
ILEUM 54
URETER 53
Iliolumbar a. & v. (brs.) 52
PSOAS MAJOR 51
Lat. femoral cutaneous n. 50
Femoral n. 49
Gluteus medius 48
ILIACUS 47
ILIUM 46
EXT. ILIAC a. & INT. ILIAC a. 45
Sympathetic trunk 44
SACROILIAC JOINT 43
COMMON ILIAC v. 42
Interosseous sacroiliac lig. 41
Sup. rectal a. & v. 40
Iliocostalis lumborum (tend.) 39
Post. longitudinal lig. 38
LUMBAR VERTEBRA V 37
Median sacral a. 36
Intervertebral disk V 35

1 ILEUM
2 Rectus Abdominis
3 Peritoneal cavity
4 Inf. epigastric a.
5 Mesentery
6 Rectus abdominis (ant. sheath)
7 ILEUM
8 Intercostal n. XII
9 Iliocolic a. & v.
10 Transversus abdominis
11 ASCENDING COLON & ext. oblique
12 Iliohypogastric n.
13 ILEUM
14 Deep circumflex iliac a. & v. & ilioinguinal n.
15 Right colic a. & v. & gluteus minimus
16 Ext. spermatic n. & spermatic a. & v.
17 URETER & ILIUM
18 Lat. femoral cutaneous n.
19 EXT. ILIAC a.
20 Int. iliac a.
21 COMMON ILIAC v. & femoral n.
22 Sympathetic trunk
23 Obturator n. & lumbar n. IV
24 SACRUM (lat. part)
25 Ant. sacroiliac lig.
26 Lumbar n. V
27 Interosseous sacroiliac lig.
28 ILIUM
29 Sacrum (sup. art. proc.)
30 Joint space
31 Lumb. vert. V (inf. art. proc.)
32 Sacral n. I
33 Multifidus & iliocostalis lumborum
34 Lig. flavum & lumbar vertebra V (spinous process)

Section 36

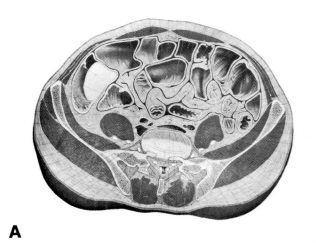

A

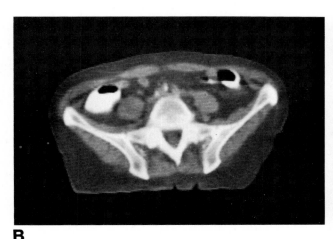

B

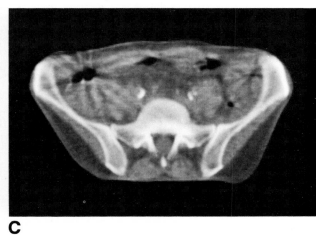

C

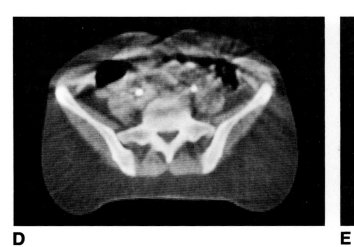

D

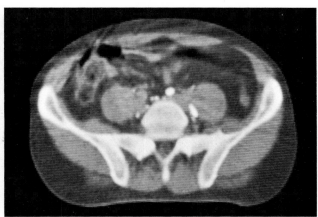

E

SECTION 36

Figure (**A**) is Section 36 reversed. The transition between L5 and S1 shows the iliac muscle (47) lying separate from the psoas (51). The gluteus medius (48) lies lateral to the iliac bone (17, 46). The iliac arteries (19, 45) are medial to the psoas (51) and easily identified when calcified (**B, C**). The ureters (17, 53) are also visible when opacified (**D**). Lymph nodes are often seen and are opacified in (**E**). The colon contains air and contrast material (**B**).

Section 36

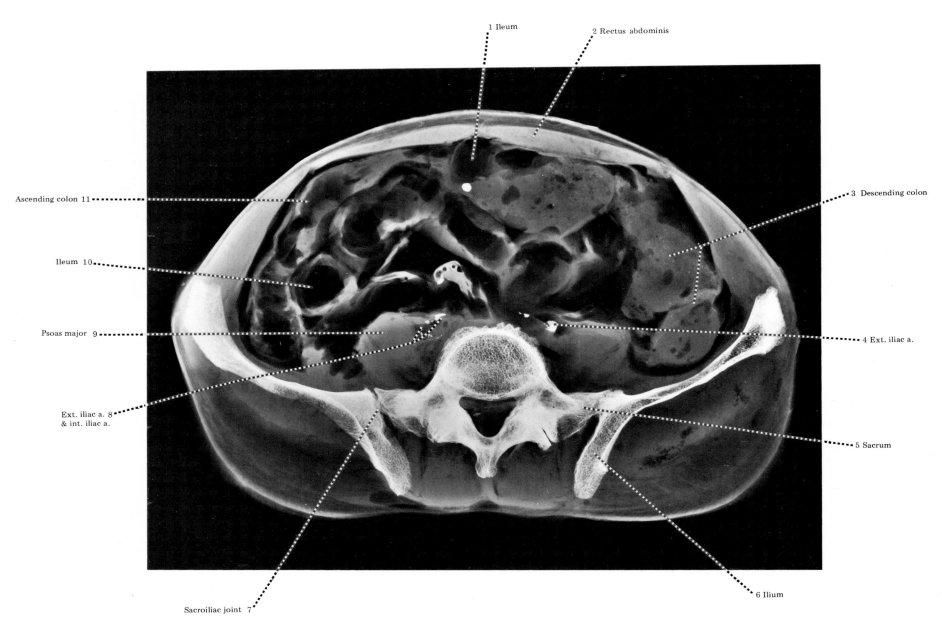

1 Ileum

2 Rectus abdominis

3 Descending colon

Ascending colon 11

Ileum 10

Psoas major 9

Ext. iliac a. 8
& int. iliac a.

4 Ext. iliac a.

5 Sacrum

6 Ilium

Sacroiliac joint 7

Section 36   (x-ray)

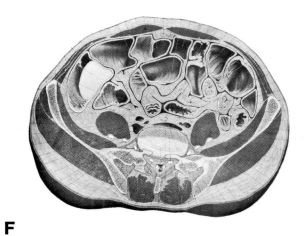

F

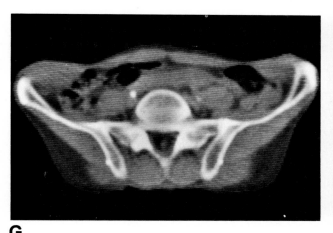

G

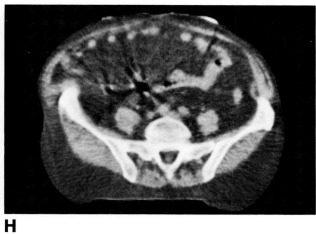

H

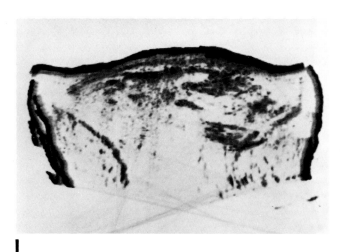

I

SECTION 36 (cont.)

Figure (**F**) is Section 36 reversed. Calcified iliac vessels (**G**-8) medial to the psoas are evident on this CT scan (**G**) of a cadaver, taken at the level of S1 (5). Air- and fluid-containing loops of bowel (1, 3, 10, 11) are visualized and in an obese person, they tend to float (**H**). Barium paste is on the skin surface.

In the echogram (**I**), the echoes from the iliac wings form a most prominent structure. On the right side, the ascending colon (11) and cecum form a major impediment to the visualization of deeper structures. However, on the left side, the thin margin of the iliac muscle is seen lying against the ilium.

Section 36

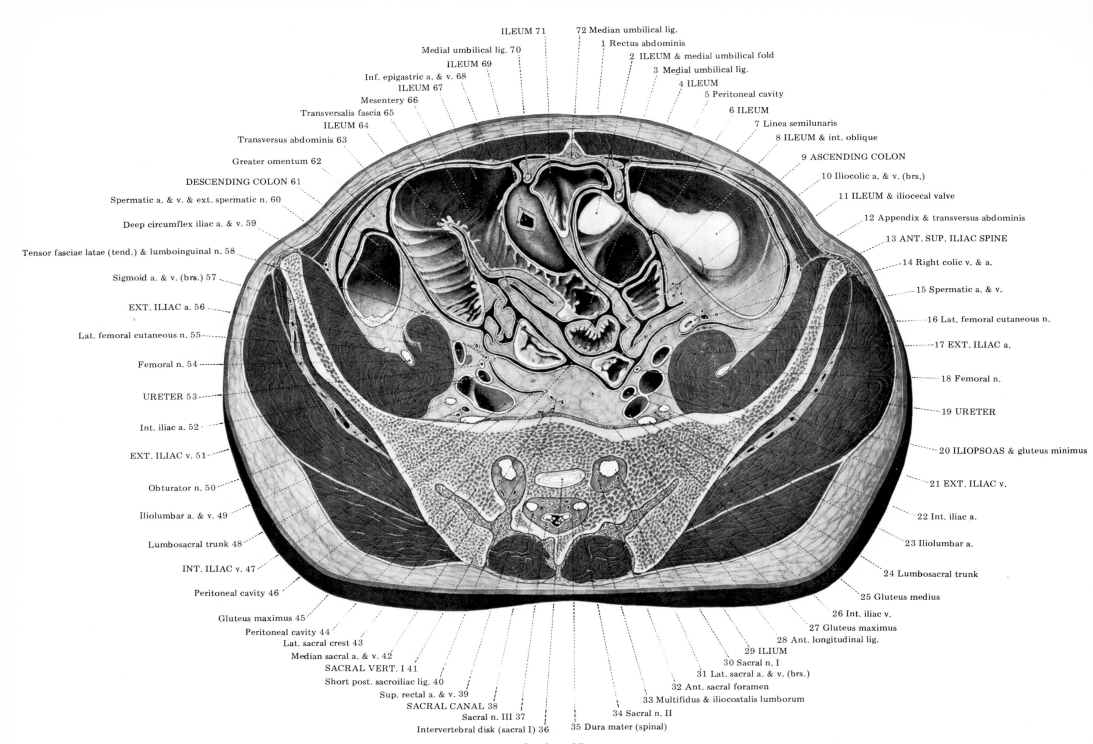

ILEUM 71   72 Median umbilical lig.

Medial umbilical lig. 70   1 Rectus abdominis

ILEUM 69   2 ILEUM & medial umbilical fold

Inf. epigastric a. & v. 68   3 Medial umbilical lig.

ILEUM 67   4 ILEUM

Mesentery 66   5 Peritoneal cavity

Transversalis fascia 65   6 ILEUM

ILEUM 64   7 Linea semilunaris

Transversus abdominis 63   8 ILEUM & int. oblique

Greater omentum 62   9 ASCENDING COLON

DESCENDING COLON 61   10 Iliocolic a. & v. (brs.)

Spermatic a. & v. & ext. spermatic n. 60   11 ILEUM & iliocecal valve

Deep circumflex iliac a. & v. 59   12 Appendix & transversus abdominis

Tensor fasciae latae (tend.) & lumboinguinal n. 58   13 ANT. SUP. ILIAC SPINE

Sigmoid a. & v. (brs.) 57   14 Right colic v. & a.

EXT. ILIAC a. 56   15 Spermatic a. & v.

Lat. femoral cutaneous n. 55   16 Lat. femoral cutaneous n.

Femoral n. 54   17 EXT. ILIAC a.

URETER 53   18 Femoral n.

Int. iliac a. 52   19 URETER

EXT. ILIAC v. 51   20 ILIOPSOAS & gluteus minimus

Obturator n. 50   21 EXT. ILIAC v.

Iliolumbar a. & v. 49   22 Int. iliac a.

Lumbosacral trunk 48   23 Iliolumbar a.

INT. ILIAC v. 47   24 Lumbosacral trunk

Peritoneal cavity 46   25 Gluteus medius

Gluteus maximus 45   26 Int. iliac v.

Peritoneal cavity 44   27 Gluteus maximus

Lat. sacral crest 43   28 Ant. longitudinal lig.

Median sacral a. & v. 42   29 ILIUM

SACRAL VERT. I 41   30 Sacral n. I

Short post. sacroiliac lig. 40   31 Lat. sacral a. & v. (brs.)

Sup. rectal a. & v. 39   32 Ant. sacral foramen

SACRAL CANAL 38   33 Multifidus & iliocostalis lumborum

Sacral n. III 37   34 Sacral n. II

Intervertebral disk (sacral I) 36   35 Dura mater (spinal)

Section 37

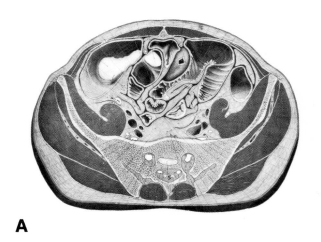

A

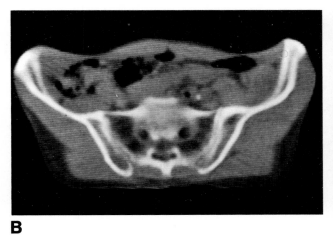

B

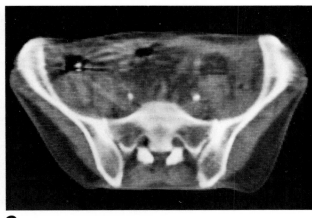

C

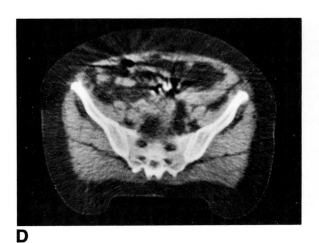

D

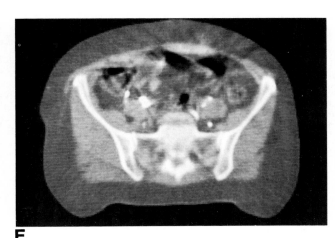

E

SECTION 37

Figure (**A**) is Section 37 reversed. The first and second sacral segments (41) and sacroiliac joints are visible at this level. The number of sacral segments seen varies with the inclination of the sacrum. The iliac bone with the anterior superior iliac spine (13) is also evident, as are the iliopsoas muscles (20). The iliac arteries (17) lie medial to this muscle and are readily identified when calcified (**B, C**). Numerous lymph nodes can be seen lying anterior, medial, and posterior to the psoas muscle (**E**). The ileum and colon contain fluid, air, and fecal material. The rectus abdominis (1) is best seen in (**B**).

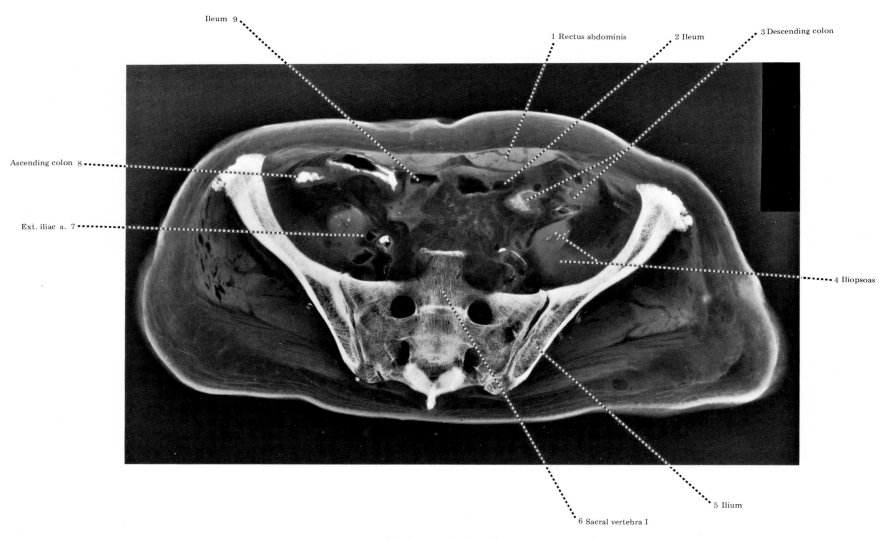

Ileum 9

1 Rectus abdominis

2 Ileum

3 Descending colon

Ascending colon 8

Ext. iliac a. 7

4 Iliopsoas

5 Ilium

6 Sacral vertebra I

Section 37 (x-ray)

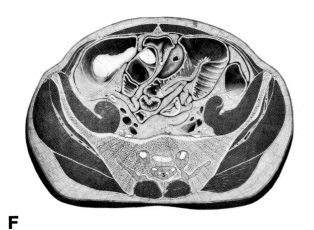

F

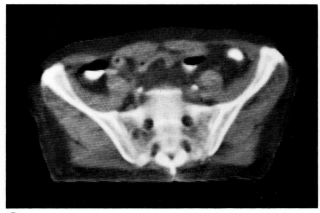

G

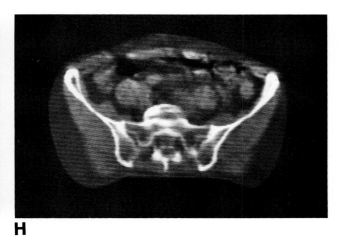

H

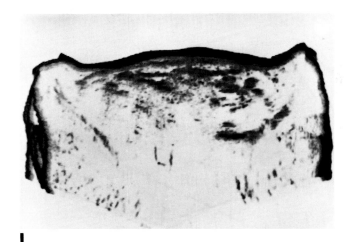

I

SECTION 37 (cont.)

Figure (**F**) is Section 37 reversed. Figure (**G**) is a CT scan of a cadaver which is similar to the specimen x-ray on the opposite page. The sacral segments (6), sacroiliac joints, iliac bone (5), and iliopsoas muscles (4) are clearly seen, as are the iliac arteries (7), which are calcified and lie just medial to the iliopsoas. A small amount of contrast material is present in the ascending (**G**-8) and descending (**G**-3) colon. The small bowel (9) contains air and fluid. Figure (**H**) shows similar findings in another patient taken at a slightly different level.

In the echogram (**I**), there is very limited visualization of abdominal structures at this level. The rectus abdominis muscles (1) are well seen. On the left side, the anterior margin of the iliac wing (5) is noted with the united iliopsoas muscles (4). The right iliac wing and sacrum (6) are only partially visualized because of the extensively gas-filled bowel.

Section 37

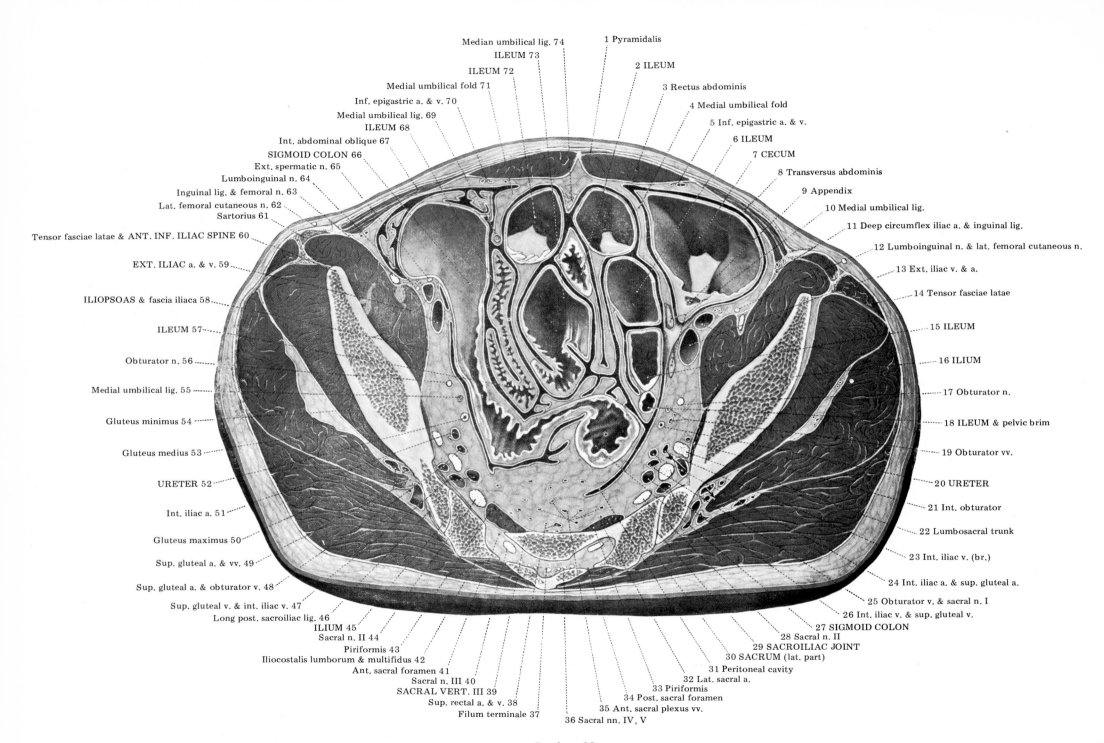

Median umbilical lig. 74
ILEUM 73
ILEUM 72
Medial umbilical fold 71
Inf. epigastric a. & v. 70
Medial umbilical lig. 69
ILEUM 68
Int. abdominal oblique 67
SIGMOID COLON 66
Ext. spermatic n. 65
Lumboinguinal n. 64
Inguinal lig. & femoral n. 63
Lat. femoral cutaneous n. 62
Sartorius 61
Tensor fasciae latae & ANT. INF. ILIAC SPINE 60
EXT. ILIAC a. & v. 59
ILIOPSOAS & fascia iliaca 58
ILEUM 57
Obturator n. 56
Medial umbilical lig. 55
Gluteus minimus 54
Gluteus medius 53
URETER 52
Int. iliac a. 51
Gluteus maximus 50
Sup. gluteal a. & vv. 49
Sup. gluteal a. & obturator v. 48
Sup. gluteal v. & int. iliac v. 47
Long post. sacroiliac lig. 46
ILIUM 45
Sacral n. II 44
Piriformis 43
Iliocostalis lumborum & multifidus 42
Ant. sacral foramen 41
Sacral n. III 40
SACRAL VERT. III 39
Sup. rectal a. & v. 38
Filum terminale 37
36 Sacral nn. IV, V

1 Pyramidalis
2 ILEUM
3 Rectus abdominis
4 Medial umbilical fold
5 Inf. epigastric a. & v.
6 ILEUM
7 CECUM
8 Transversus abdominis
9 Appendix
10 Medial umbilical lig.
11 Deep circumflex iliac a. & inguinal lig.
12 Lumboinguinal n. & lat. femoral cutaneous n.
13 Ext. iliac v. & a.
14 Tensor fasciae latae
15 ILEUM
16 ILIUM
17 Obturator n.
18 ILEUM & pelvic brim
19 Obturator vv.
20 URETER
21 Int. obturator
22 Lumbosacral trunk
23 Int. iliac v. (br.)
24 Int. iliac a. & sup. gluteal a.
25 Obturator v. & sacral n. I
26 Int. iliac v. & sup. gluteal v.
27 SIGMOID COLON
28 Sacral n. II
29 SACROILIAC JOINT
30 SACRUM (lat. part)
31 Peritoneal cavity
32 Lat. sacral a.
33 Piriformis
34 Post. sacral foramen
35 Ant. sacral plexus vv.

Section 38

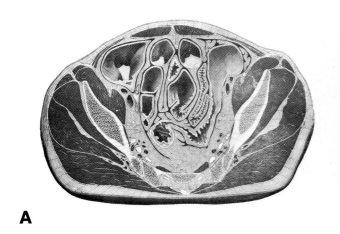

A

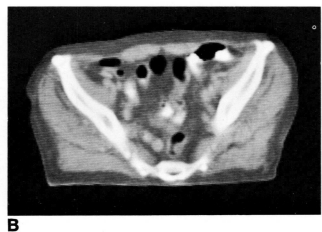

B

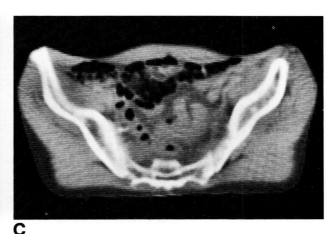

C

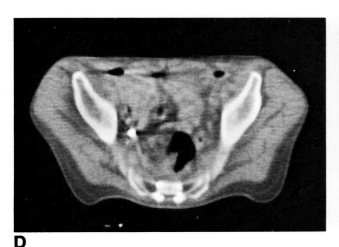

D

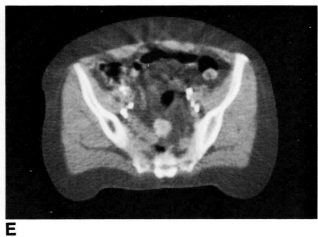

E

SECTION 38

Figure (**A**) is Section 38 reversed. At the level of S3 (39) the inferior portion of the sacroiliac joint is seen. The sigmoid colon (27) and cecum (7) may be seen containing some contrast material (**B**), and loops of ileum (72) are seen which contain air and fluid. The iliopsoas muscle (58) is medial to the iliac bone (16), and the gluteus maximus (50), gluteus medius (53), and gluteus minimus (54) are all evident. Some lymph nodes have been opacified (**E**) by lymphangiography which shows their position relative to the iliopsoas (58). A calcified node is present in (**D**). The rectus abdominis muscle is readily seen (**B**-3).

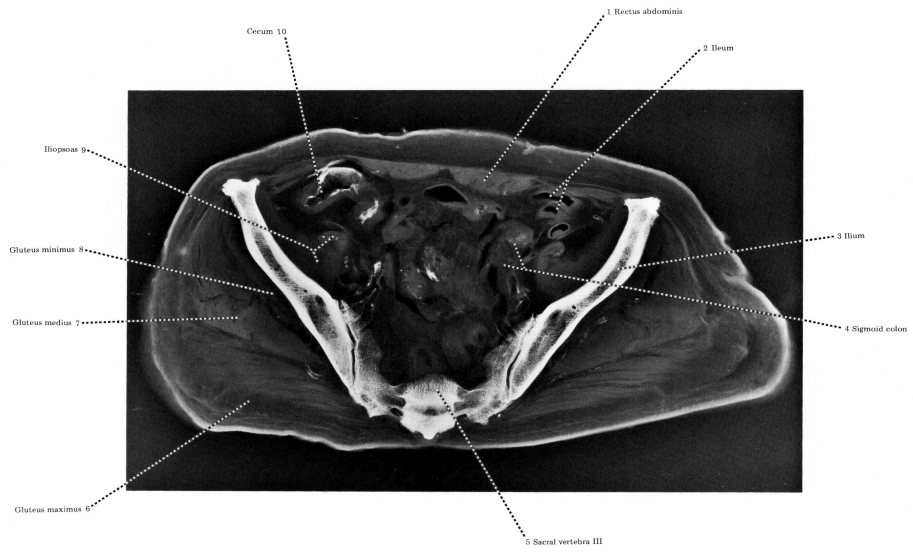

Cecum 10

1 Rectus abdominis

2 Ileum

Iliopsoas 9

3 Ilium

Gluteus minimus 8

Gluteus medius 7

4 Sigmoid colon

Gluteus maximus 6

5 Sacral vertebra III

Section 38 (x-ray)

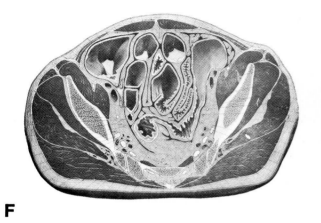

F

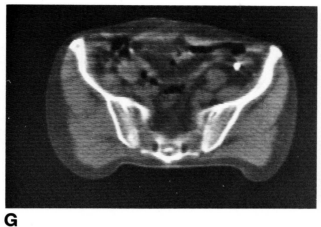

G

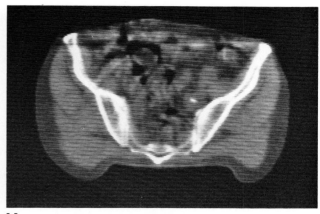

H

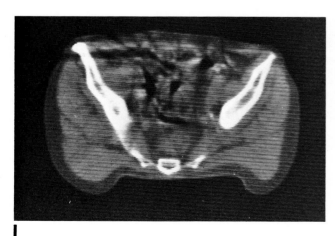

I

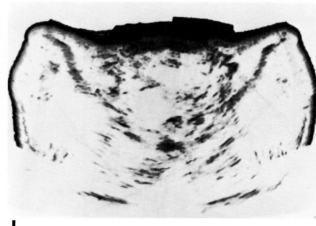

J

SECTION 38 (cont.)

Figure (**F**) is Section 38 reversed. CT scans (**G**), (**H**), and (**I**) show numerous loops of bowel within the pelvis, containing air and fluid, and these represent primarily the ileum (2), the sigmoid (4), and the cecum (10). The iliopsoas muscle (9) is just medial to the ilium (3), whereas the gluteal muscles (6, 7, 8) lie laterally. The section is taken through the level of S3 (5). Calcified lymph nodes are visible in the CT scans taken of this patient at slightly different levels.

In the echogram (**J**), the more anteriorly situated iliopsoas muscles (9) now form a more clearly defined anatomic landmark just anteromedial to the iliac bones (3). The iliac artery and vein can be defined just medial to the iliopsoas. Midline structures are still obscured by extensive bowel gas.

Section 38

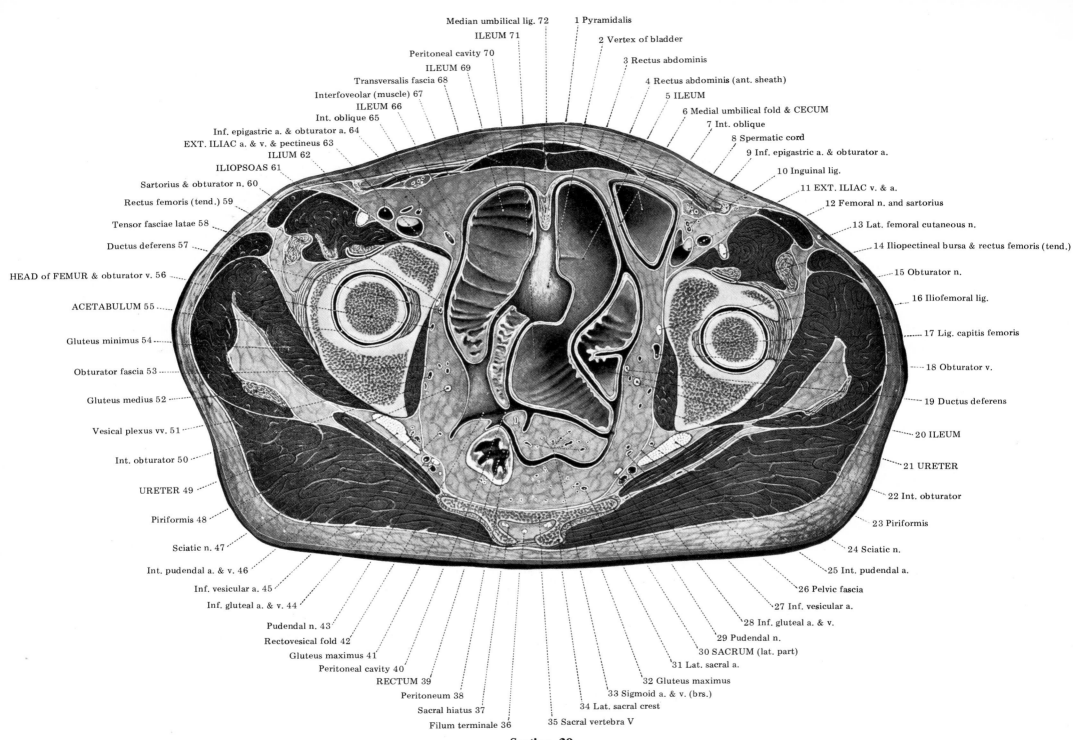

Median umbilical lig. 72
ILEUM 71
Peritoneal cavity 70
ILEUM 69
Transversalis fascia 68
Interfoveolar (muscle) 67
ILEUM 66
Int. oblique 65
Inf. epigastric a. & obturator a. 64
EXT. ILIAC a. & v. & pectineus 63
ILIUM 62
ILIOPSOAS 61
Sartorius & obturator n. 60
Rectus femoris (tend.) 59
Tensor fasciae latae 58
Ductus deferens 57
HEAD of FEMUR & obturator v. 56
ACETABULUM 55
Gluteus minimus 54
Obturator fascia 53
Gluteus medius 52
Vesical plexus vv. 51
Int. obturator 50
URETER 49
Piriformis 48
Sciatic n. 47
Int. pudendal a. & v. 46
Inf. vesicular a. 45
Inf. gluteal a. & v. 44
Pudendal n. 43
Rectovesical fold 42
Gluteus maximus 41
Peritoneal cavity 40
RECTUM 39
Peritoneum 38
Sacral hiatus 37
Filum terminale 36

1 Pyramidalis
2 Vertex of bladder
3 Rectus abdominis
4 Rectus abdominis (ant. sheath)
5 ILEUM
6 Medial umbilical fold & CECUM
7 Int. oblique
8 Spermatic cord
9 Inf. epigastric a. & obturator a.
10 Inguinal lig.
11 EXT. ILIAC v. & a.
12 Femoral n. and sartorius
13 Lat. femoral cutaneous n.
14 Iliopectineal bursa & rectus femoris (tend.)
15 Obturator n.
16 Iliofemoral lig.
17 Lig. capitis femoris
18 Obturator v.
19 Ductus deferens
20 ILEUM
21 URETER
22 Int. obturator
23 Piriformis
24 Sciatic n.
25 Int. pudendal a.
26 Pelvic fascia
27 Inf. vesicular a.
28 Inf. gluteal a. & v.
29 Pudendal n.
30 SACRUM (lat. part)
31 Lat. sacral a.
32 Gluteus maximus
33 Sigmoid a. & v. (brs.)
34 Lat. sacral crest
35 Sacral vertebra V

Section 39

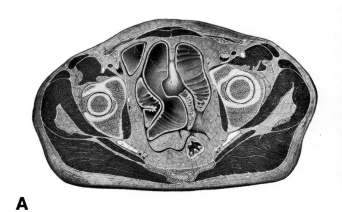

A

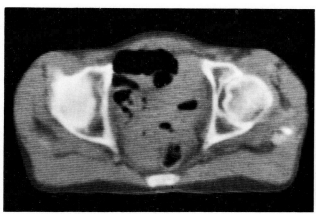

B

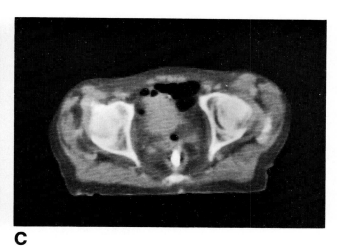

C

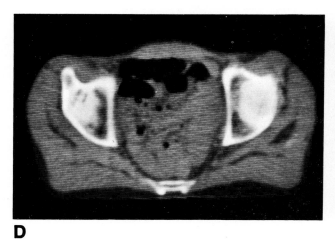

D

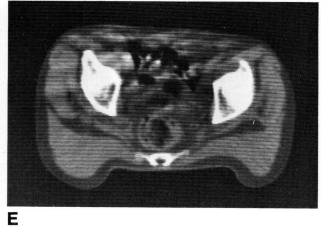

E

SECTION 39

Figure (**A**) is Section 39 reversed. This section through the acetabulum (55) and the 5th sacral segment (35) shows the ileum (5) and rectum (39) containing fluid and air. A notch for the ligamentum teres (**B**-17) may be seen in the femoral head. The external iliac vessels (11) are medial to the iliopsoas (61) which is anterior to the iliac bone (62). The rectus abdominis muscles (3) are seen anteriorly. Contrast material is present in the rectum (**C**-39).

Section 39

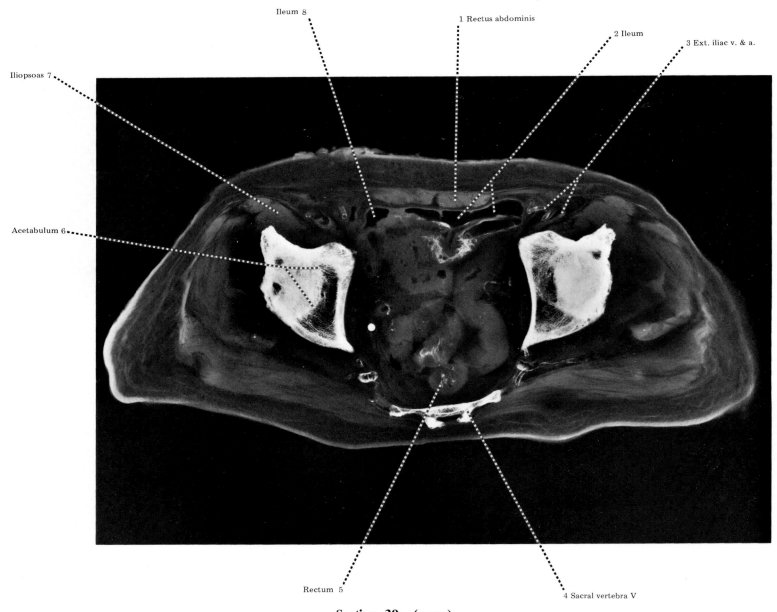

Ileum 8

1 Rectus abdominis

2 Ileum

3 Ext. iliac v. & a.

Iliopsoas 7

Acetabulum 6

Rectum 5

4 Sacral vertebra V

Section 39 (x-ray)

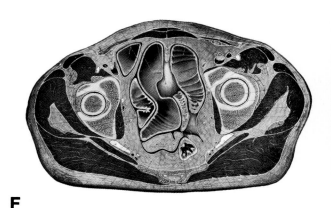

F

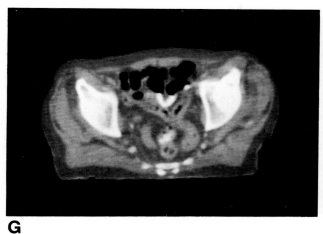

G

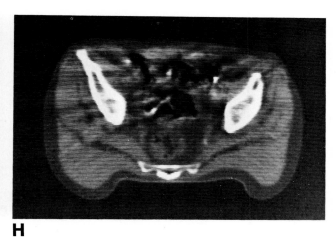

H

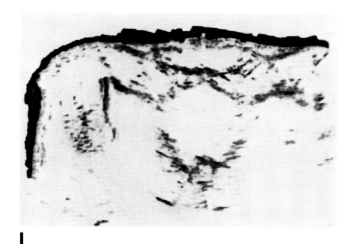

I

SECTION 39 (cont.)

Figure (**F**) is Section 39 reversed. A CT scan (**G**) taken of a cadaver which was subsequently sectioned (opposite page) shows many fluid-filled and air-containing loops of ileum (2) within the pelvis at the level of the acetabulum (6). The rectum (5) is anterior to the sacrum (4), and the external iliac vessels (3) are medial to the iliopsoas (7).

In the echogram (**I**), the more transversely situated osseous margins of the pelvis overlying the acetabulum (6) are now seen. The iliopsoas muscle (7) is correspondingly flattened and located more laterally. The external iliac artery and vein (3) can be identified on the right side. The anterior echo-free area probably represents the upper portion of a urine-filled bladder.

Section 39

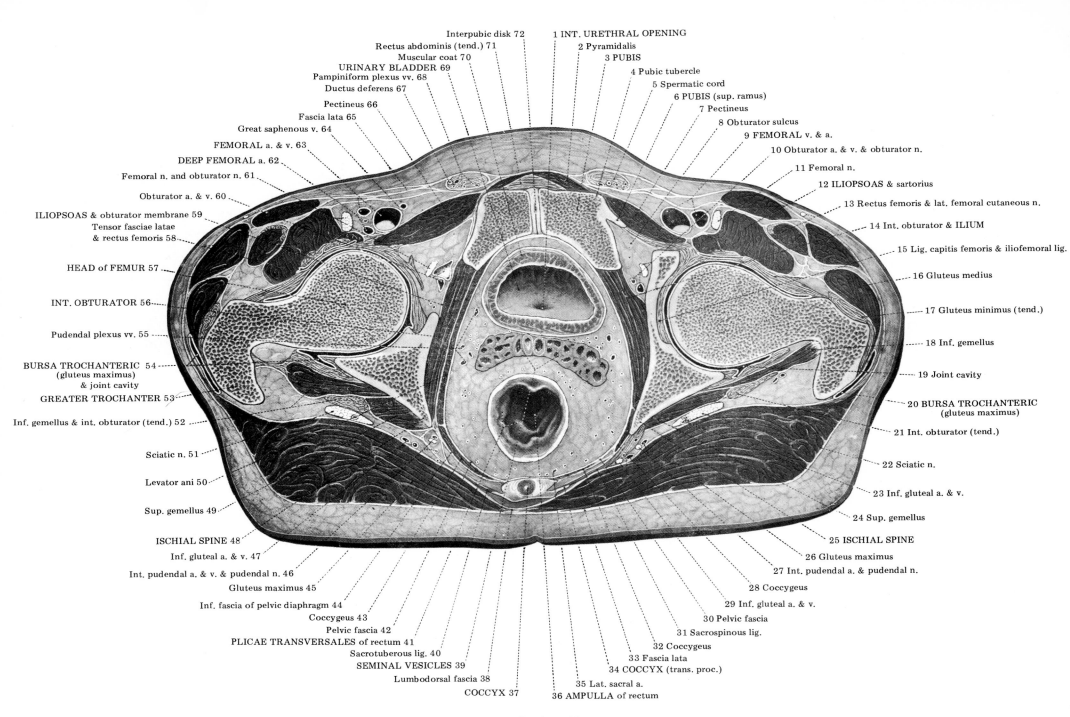

Interpubic disk 72
Rectus abdominis (tend.) 71
Muscular coat 70
URINARY BLADDER 69
Pampiniform plexus vv. 68
Ductus deferens 67
Pectineus 66
Fascia lata 65
Great saphenous v. 64
FEMORAL a. & v. 63
DEEP FEMORAL a. 62
Femoral n. and obturator n. 61
Obturator a. & v. 60
ILIOPSOAS & obturator membrane 59
Tensor fasciae latae
& rectus femoris 58
HEAD of FEMUR 57
INT. OBTURATOR 56
Pudendal plexus vv. 55
BURSA TROCHANTERIC 54
(gluteus maximus)
& joint cavity
GREATER TROCHANTER 53
Inf. gemellus & int. obturator (tend.) 52
Sciatic n. 51
Levator ani 50
Sup. gemellus 49
ISCHIAL SPINE 48
Inf. gluteal a. & v. 47
Int. pudendal a. & v. & pudendal n. 46
Gluteus maximus 45
Inf. fascia of pelvic diaphragm 44
Coccygeus 43
Pelvic fascia 42
PLICAE TRANSVERSALES of rectum 41
Sacrotuberous lig. 40
SEMINAL VESICLES 39
Lumbodorsal fascia 38
COCCYX 37

1 INT. URETHRAL OPENING
2 Pyramidalis
3 PUBIS
4 Pubic tubercle
5 Spermatic cord
6 PUBIS (sup. ramus)
7 Pectineus
8 Obturator sulcus
9 FEMORAL v. & a.
10 Obturator a. & v. & obturator n.
11 Femoral n.
12 ILIOPSOAS & sartorius
13 Rectus femoris & lat. femoral cutaneous n.
14 Int. obturator & ILIUM
15 Lig. capitis femoris & iliofemoral lig.
16 Gluteus medius
17 Gluteus minimus (tend.)
18 Inf. gemellus
19 Joint cavity
20 BURSA TROCHANTERIC
(gluteus maximus)
21 Int. obturator (tend.)
22 Sciatic n.
23 Inf. gluteal a. & v.
24 Sup. gemellus
25 ISCHIAL SPINE
26 Gluteus maximus
27 Int. pudendal a. & pudendal n.
28 Coccygeus
29 Inf. gluteal a. & v.
30 Pelvic fascia
31 Sacrospinous lig.
32 Coccygeus
33 Fascia lata
34 COCCYX (trans. proc.)
35 Lat. sacral a.
36 AMPULLA of rectum

Section 40

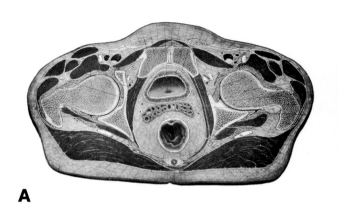

A

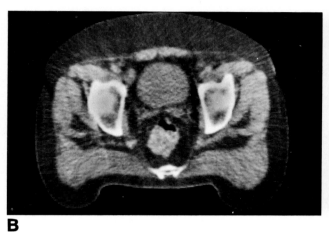

B

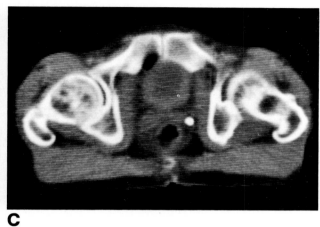

C

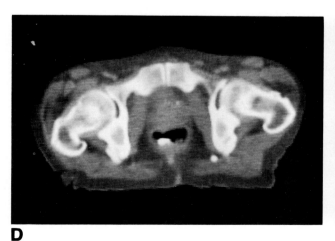

D

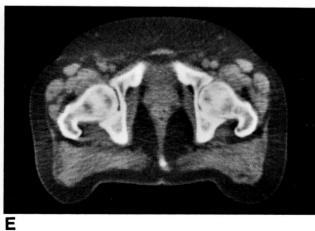

E

SECTION 40

Figure (**A**) is Section 40 reversed. The CT scans are shown at slightly different levels because of patient variation. The seminal vesicles (39), which lie posterior to the bladder (69), are anterior to the rectum (36), as shown in (**B**). The floor of the bladder and the prostate are evident slightly caudad (**D, E**), as shown in the x-ray of the specimen (next page) and in Section 41. The obturator internus (14) passes from the pubis, inferior to the ischial spine (25) laterally to insert on the femur. The fascia and muscles of the pelvic diaphragm (44) are seen (**D, E**). The ischial spine (**E**-25), acetabulum, femoral head (57), and greater trochanter (53) are also evident. The femoral vessels (9) are medial to the iliopsoas muscle (12). The spermatic cord (5) lies anterolateral to the pubic bone (3) and is seen in (**C, D**).

Section 40

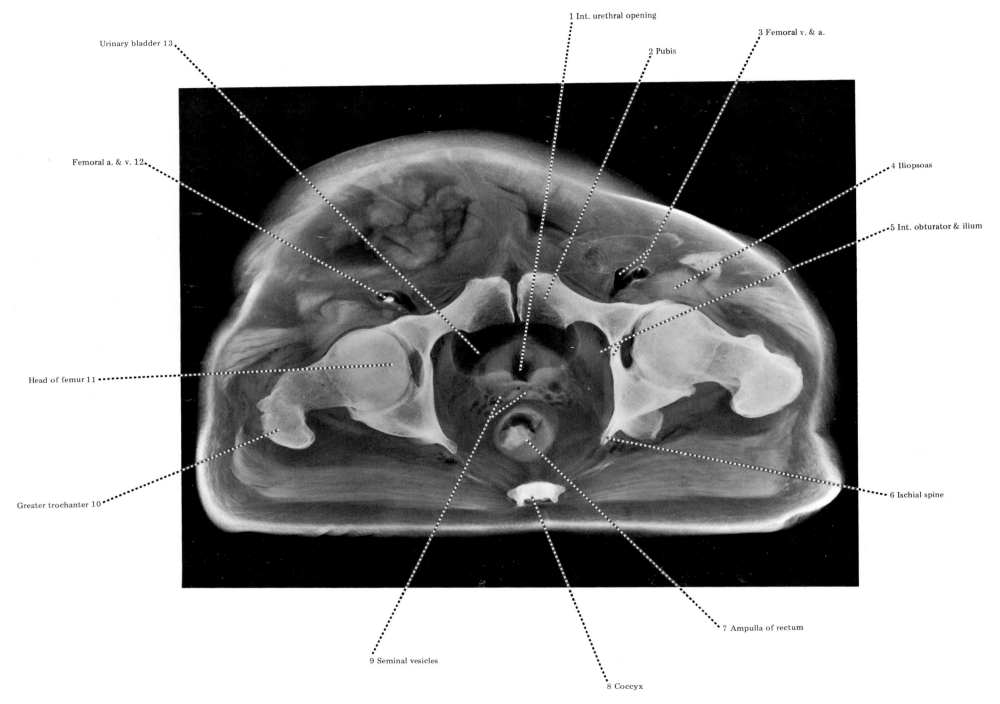

1 Int. urethral opening

2 Pubis

3 Femoral v. & a.

Urinary bladder 13

Femoral a. & v. 12

4 Iliopsoas

5 Int. obturator & ilium

Head of femur 11

6 Ischial spine

Greater trochanter 10

7 Ampulla of rectum

9 Seminal vesicles

8 Coccyx

Section 40 (x-ray)

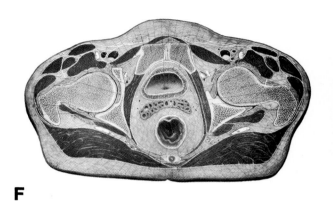

F

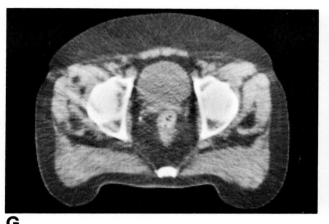

G

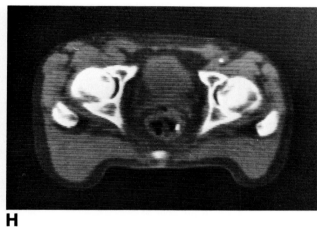

H

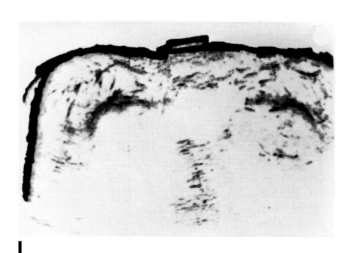

I

SECTION 40 (cont.)

Figure (**F**) is Section 40 reversed. CT scans (**G, H**) taken slightly cephalad to the x-ray of the specimen (opposite page) show the bladder (13) containing urine, although the bladder contains air in the specimen. The seminal vesicles (9) are between the bladder (13) and rectum (7). The ischial spine (6), coccyx (8), inferior pelvic diaphragm, femoral head (11), and greater trochanter (10) are also visible. The femoral vessels (3) have calcified walls and lie medial to the iliopsoas (4).

In the echogram (**I**), the iliopsoas (4) and other anterior and lateral muscles of the upper thigh are now well shown. The bladder (13) can be seen in the midline, but is partly obscured by the symphysis pubis (2) anteriorly. The rounded structure of the acetabulum presents a very strong, characteristic echo.

Section 40

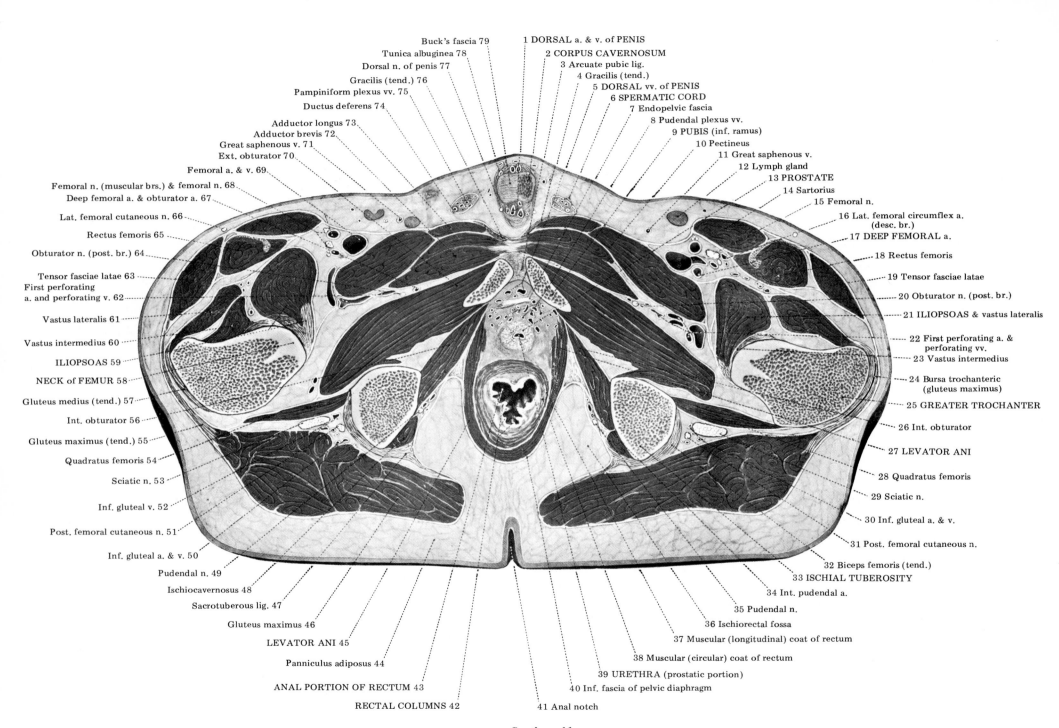

Buck's fascia 79
Tunica albuginea 78
Dorsal n. of penis 77
Gracilis (tend.) 76
Pampiniform plexus vv. 75
Ductus deferens 74
Adductor longus 73
Adductor brevis 72
Great saphenous v. 71
Ext. obturator 70
Femoral a. & v. 69
Femoral n. (muscular brs.) & femoral n. 68
Deep femoral a. & obturator a. 67
Lat. femoral cutaneous n. 66
Rectus femoris 65
Obturator n. (post. br.) 64
Tensor fasciae latae 63
First perforating
a. and perforating v. 62
Vastus lateralis 61
Vastus intermedius 60
ILIOPSOAS 59
NECK of FEMUR 58
Gluteus medius (tend.) 57
Int. obturator 56
Gluteus maximus (tend.) 55
Quadratus femoris 54
Sciatic n. 53
Inf. gluteal v. 52
Post. femoral cutaneous n. 51
Inf. gluteal a. & v. 50
Pudendal n. 49
Ischiocavernosus 48
Sacrotuberous lig. 47
Gluteus maximus 46
LEVATOR ANI 45
Panniculus adiposus 44
ANAL PORTION OF RECTUM 43
RECTAL COLUMNS 42

1 DORSAL a. & v. of PENIS
2 CORPUS CAVERNOSUM
3 Arcuate pubic lig.
4 Gracilis (tend.)
5 DORSAL vv. of PENIS
6 SPERMATIC CORD
7 Endopelvic fascia
8 Pudendal plexus vv.
9 PUBIS (inf. ramus)
10 Pectineus
11 Great saphenous v.
12 Lymph gland
13 PROSTATE
14 Sartorius
15 Femoral n.
16 Lat. femoral circumflex a.
(desc. br.)
17 DEEP FEMORAL a.
18 Rectus femoris
19 Tensor fasciae latae
20 Obturator n. (post. br.)
21 ILIOPSOAS & vastus lateralis
22 First perforating a. &
perforating vv.
23 Vastus intermedius
24 Bursa trochanteric
(gluteus maximus)
25 GREATER TROCHANTER
26 Int. obturator
27 LEVATOR ANI
28 Quadratus femoris
29 Sciatic n.
30 Inf. gluteal a. & v.
31 Post. femoral cutaneous n.
32 Biceps femoris (tend.)
33 ISCHIAL TUBEROSITY
34 Int. pudendal a.
35 Pudendal n.
36 Ischiorectal fossa
37 Muscular (longitudinal) coat of rectum
38 Muscular (circular) coat of rectum
39 URETHRA (prostatic portion)
40 Inf. fascia of pelvic diaphragm
41 Anal notch

Section 41

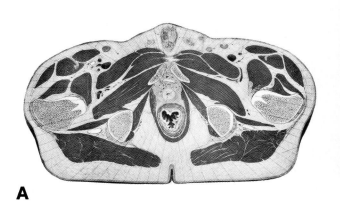

A

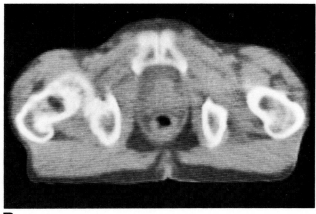

B

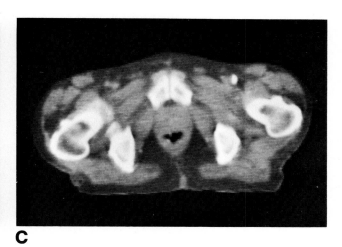

C

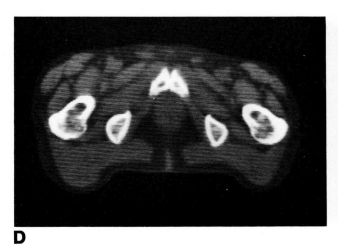

D

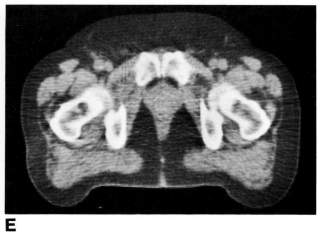

E

SECTION 41

Figure (**A**) is Section 41 reversed. The prostate (13) and pudendal plexus (8) are seen at the level of the symphysis pubis, just anterior to the rectum (43). They are enclosed by the levator ani sling (45). The internal obturator muscle (26) extends from the ischial tuberosity (33) to the pubic bone (9). Also note the ischiorectal fossa (36), femoral vessels (69), anteromedial to the iliopsoas (59), the neck of the femur (58), and spermatic cord (6). Lymph nodes may be seen in the femoral area (12).

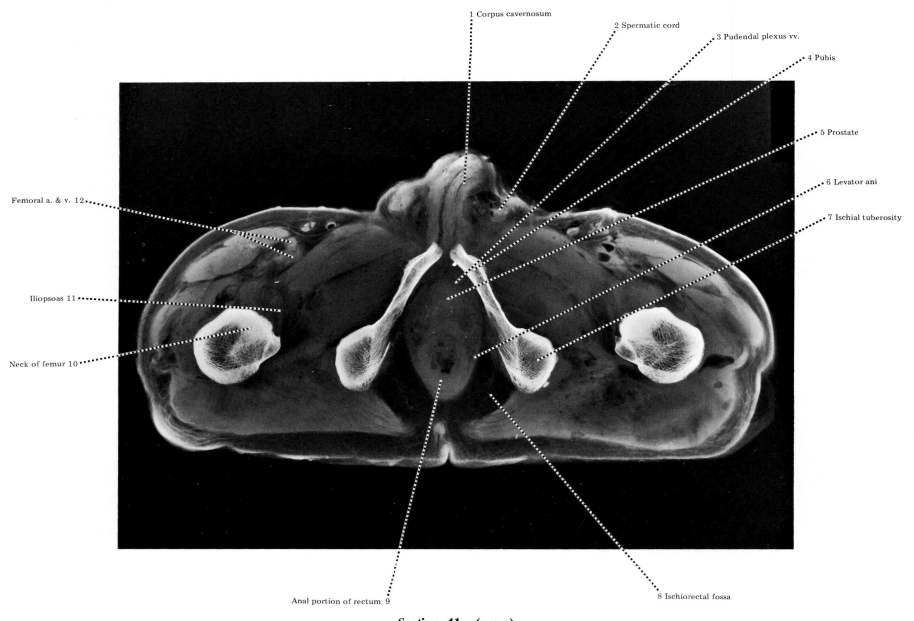

1 Corpus cavernosum

2 Spermatic cord

3 Pudendal plexus vv.

4 Pubis

5 Prostate

6 Levator ani

7 Ischial tuberosity

Femoral a. & v. 12

Iliopsoas 11

Neck of femur 10

Anal portion of rectum 9

8 Ischiorectal fossa

Section 41 (x-ray)

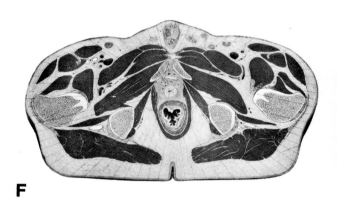

F

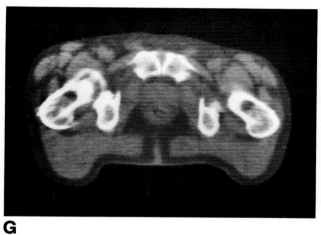

G

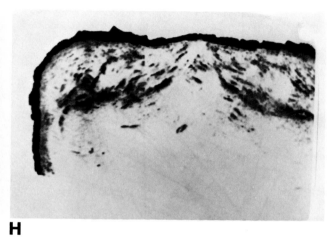

H

SECTION 41 (cont.)

Figure (**F**) is Section 41 reversed. The CT scan of a patient is very similar to the x-ray of a specimen (opposite page) taken at the level of the prostate (5) just inferior to the symphysis pubis. The levator ani (6) can be seen surrounding the rectum (9), pudendal plexus (3), and prostate (5). The spermatic cord (2) is lateral to the penis. The femoral vessels (12) are anteromedial to the iliopsoas, which is immediately anterior to the femoral neck (10).

In the echogram (**H**), while the pubic ramus (4) still obscures the anterior midline structures, the obturator externus muscle presents a characteristic oblique echo extending laterally. Some of the remaining anterior muscle groups of the thigh and pelvis can also be identified at this level.

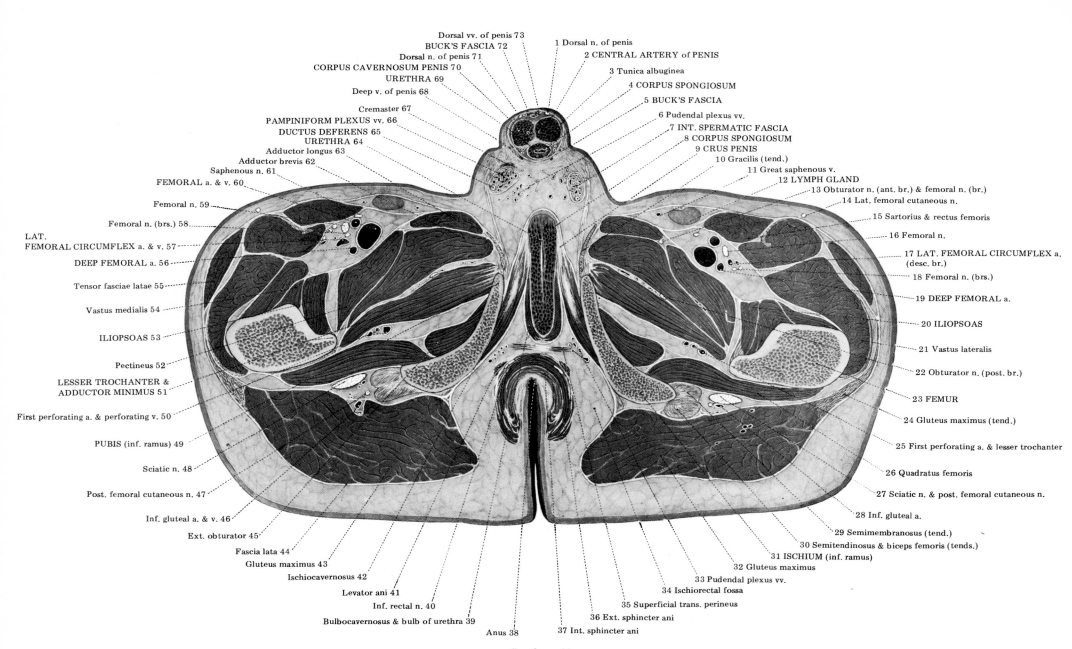

Dorsal vv. of penis 73
BUCK'S FASCIA 72
Dorsal n. of penis 71
CORPUS CAVERNOSUM PENIS 70
URETHRA 69
Deep v. of penis 68
Cremaster 67
PAMPINIFORM PLEXUS vv. 66
DUCTUS DEFERENS 65
URETHRA 64
Adductor longus 63
Adductor brevis 62
Saphenous n. 61
FEMORAL a. & v. 60
Femoral n. 59
Femoral n. (brs.) 58
LAT.
FEMORAL CIRCUMFLEX a. & v. 57
DEEP FEMORAL a. 56
Tensor fasciae latae 55
Vastus medialis 54
ILIOPSOAS 53
Pectineus 52
LESSER TROCHANTER &
ADDUCTOR MINIMUS 51
First perforating a. & perforating v. 50
PUBIS (inf. ramus) 49
Sciatic n. 48
Post. femoral cutaneous n. 47
Inf. gluteal a. & v. 46
Ext. obturator 45
Fascia lata 44
Gluteus maximus 43
Ischiocavernosus 42
Levator ani 41
Inf. rectal n. 40
Bulbocavernosus & bulb of urethra 39
Anus 38

1 Dorsal n. of penis
2 CENTRAL ARTERY of PENIS
3 Tunica albuginea
4 CORPUS SPONGIOSUM
5 BUCK'S FASCIA
6 Pudendal plexus vv.
7 INT. SPERMATIC FASCIA
8 CORPUS SPONGIOSUM
9 CRUS PENIS
10 Gracilis (tend.)
11 Great saphenous v.
12 LYMPH GLAND
13 Obturator n. (ant. br.) & femoral n. (br.)
14 Lat. femoral cutaneous n.
15 Sartorius & rectus femoris
16 Femoral n.
17 LAT. FEMORAL CIRCUMFLEX a.
(desc. br.)
18 Femoral n. (brs.)
19 DEEP FEMORAL a.
20 ILIOPSOAS
21 Vastus lateralis
22 Obturator n. (post. br.)
23 FEMUR
24 Gluteus maximus (tend.)
25 First perforating a. & lesser trochanter
26 Quadratus femoris
27 Sciatic n. & post. femoral cutaneous n.
28 Inf. gluteal a.
29 Semimembranosus (tend.)
30 Semitendinosus & biceps femoris (tends.)
31 ISCHIUM (inf. ramus)
32 Gluteus maximus
33 Pudendal plexus vv.
34 Ischiorectal fossa
35 Superficial trans. perineus
36 Ext. sphincter ani
37 Int. sphincter ani

Section 42

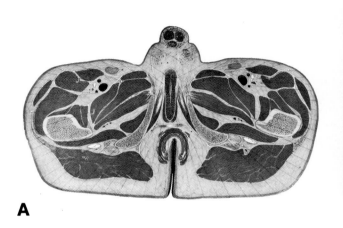

A

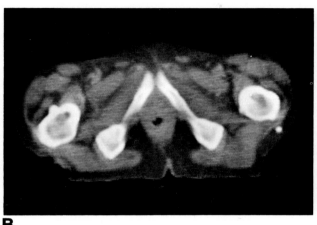

B

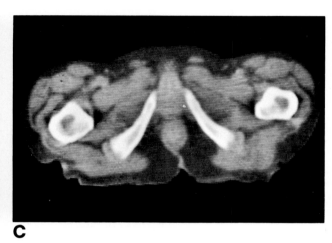

C

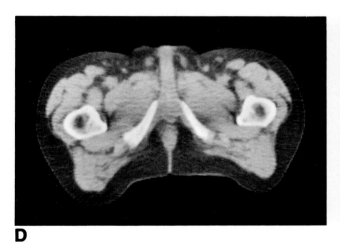

D

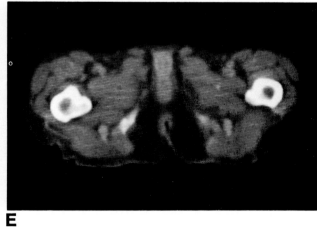

E

SECTION 42

Figure (**A**) is Section 42 reversed. These scans taken at slightly different levels in different patients show the corpus spongiosum (8) and bulbocavernosus at the level of the inferior ischial ramus (31) and inferior pubic ramus (49). The spermatic cord (65), femoral vessels (60), and nodes are seen anteriorly, whereas the anus (38) lies posteriorly within the ischiorectal fossa (34). Note the various muscles: iliopsoas (53) inserted on the lesser trochanter (51), the vastus lateralis (21) lateral to the femur (23), the quadratus femoris (26), and the gluteus maximus (32).

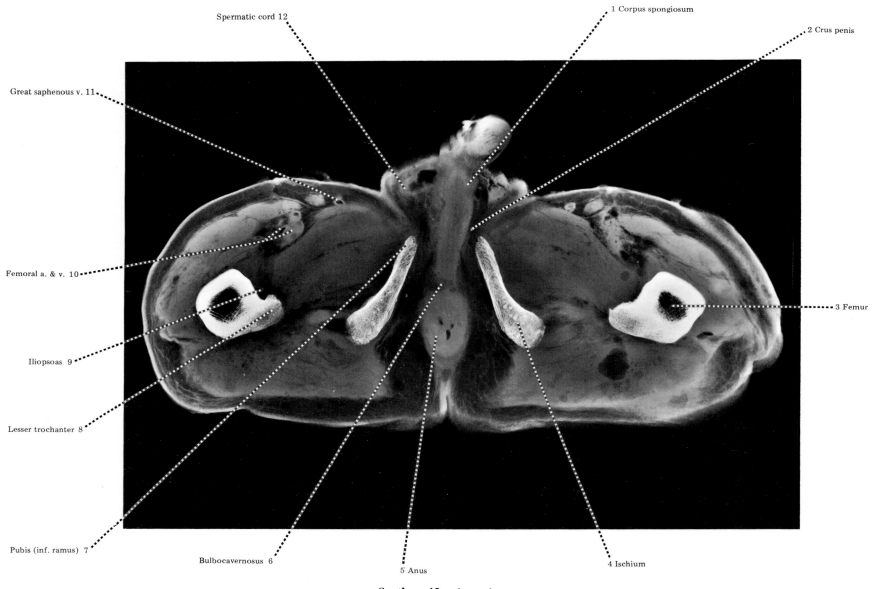

Spermatic cord 12

1 Corpus spongiosum

2 Crus penis

Great saphenous v. 11

Femoral a. & v. 10

3 Femur

Iliopsoas 9

Lesser trochanter 8

Pubis (inf. ramus) 7

Bulbocavernosus 6

5 Anus

4 Ischium

Section 42 (x-ray)

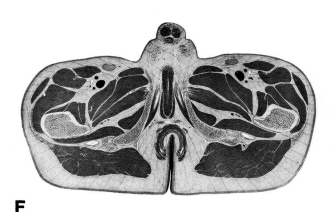

F

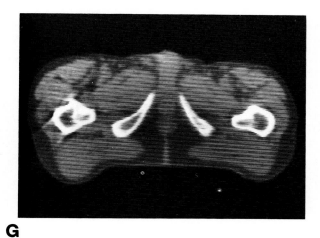

G

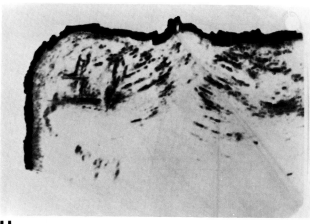

H

SECTION 42 (cont.)

Figure (**F**) is Section 42 reversed. A scan of a patient (**G**) at the same level as the cross-section of a cadaver (opposite page) shows the corpus spongiosum (1), bulbocavernosus (6), spermatic cord (12), and anus (5). The femur is sectioned at the level of the lesser trochanter (8), showing the insertion of the iliopsoas (9). The femoral vessels (10) and nodes are anteromedial to the iliopsoas.

In the echogram (**H**), the considerable muscle mass allows visualization down to the characteristic echo of the inferior ramus of the pubis (7). The oblique echoes of the obturator externus, quadratus femoris, and adductor minimus muscles can be seen. The region of the femoral artery and vein (10) can also be identified anteriorly.

Section 42

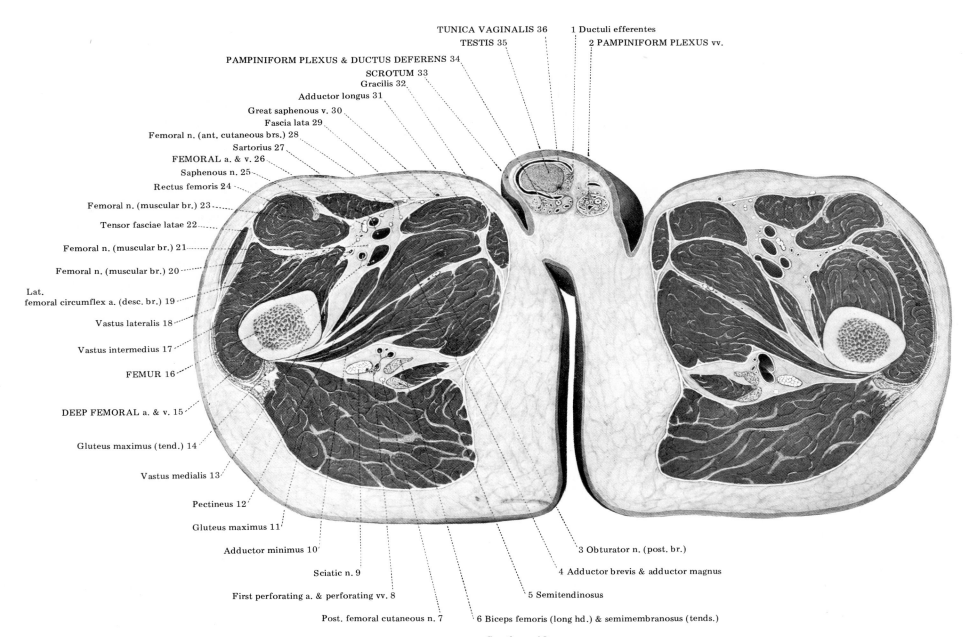

TUNICA VAGINALIS 36

TESTIS 35

PAMPINIFORM PLEXUS & DUCTUS DEFERENS 34

SCROTUM 33

Gracilis 32

Adductor longus 31

Great saphenous v. 30

Fascia lata 29

Femoral n. (ant. cutaneous brs.) 28

Sartorius 27

FEMORAL a. & v. 26

Saphenous n. 25

Rectus femoris 24

Femoral n. (muscular br.) 23

Tensor fasciae latae 22

Femoral n. (muscular br.) 21

Femoral n. (muscular br.) 20

Lat.
femoral circumflex a. (desc. br.) 19

Vastus lateralis 18

Vastus intermedius 17

FEMUR 16

DEEP FEMORAL a. & v. 15

Gluteus maximus (tend.) 14

Vastus medialis 13

Pectineus 12

Gluteus maximus 11

Adductor minimus 10

Sciatic n. 9

First perforating a. & perforating vv. 8

Post. femoral cutaneous n. 7

1 Ductuli efferentes

2 PAMPINIFORM PLEXUS vv.

3 Obturator n. (post. br.)

4 Adductor brevis & adductor magnus

5 Semitendinosus

6 Biceps femoris (long hd.) & semimembranosus (tends.)

Section 43

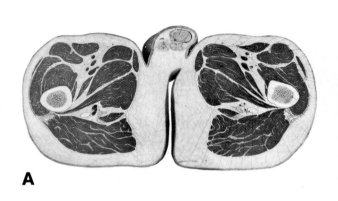

A

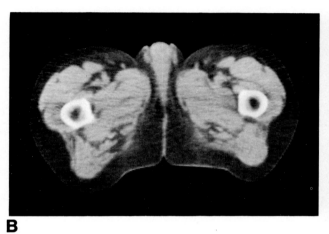

B

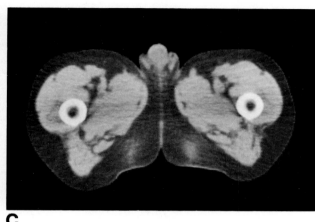

C

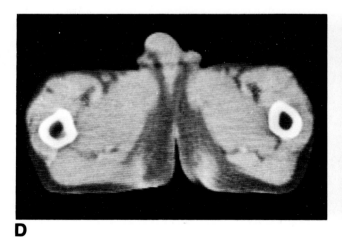

D

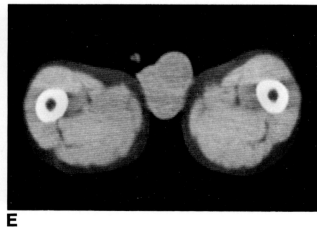

E

SECTION 43

Figure (**A**) is Section 43 reversed. Four CT scans at slightly different levels show the pampiniform plexus (2) lateral to the cavernous urethra. The scrotum (33) is seen in Figure (**E**). The femoral vessels (26) are slightly anterior to the muscles of the leg, and the femur (16) is seen across its horizontal section.

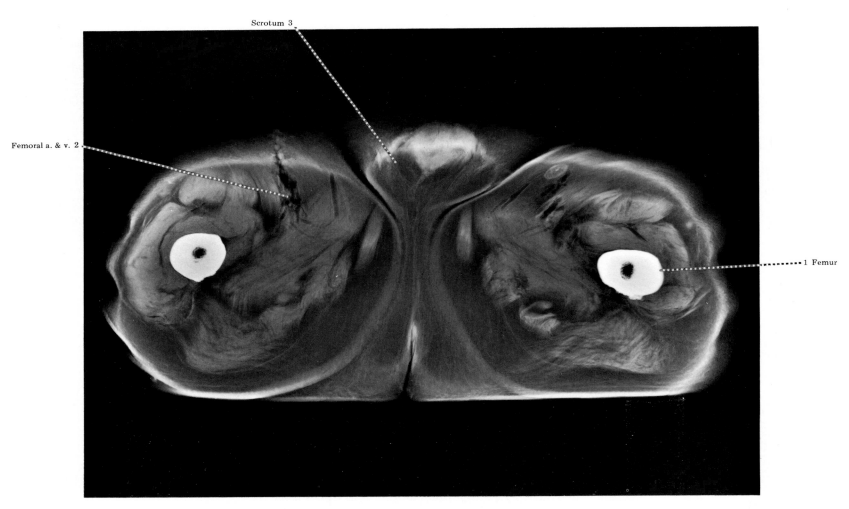

Scrotum 3

Femoral a. & v. 2

1 Femur

Section 43   (x-ray)

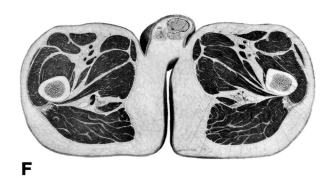

F

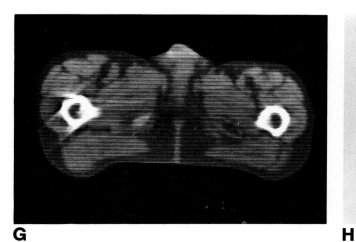

G

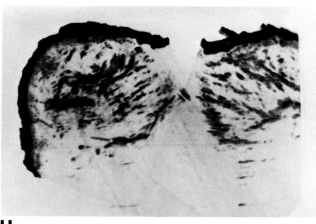

H

SECTION 43 (cont.)

Figure (**F**) is Section 43 reversed. A scan (**G**) taken through the cavernous urethra and scrotum (3) is just below the floor of the pelvis. Both femurs (1) are seen end-on, and the muscles of the thigh are sharply defined.

In the echogram (**H**), only the right thigh is completely shown in this view. The muscle groups anterior to the plane of the femur are fairly well shown, with the vastus lateralis and medius muscles and rectus femoris muscle particularly apparent.

Section 43

KEY FIGURE IX This key figure was made by replacing the Sections 44 to 48 in their normal relations and cutting them in the mesial sagittal plane. The sections included in this series show the more important structures of the female pelvis.

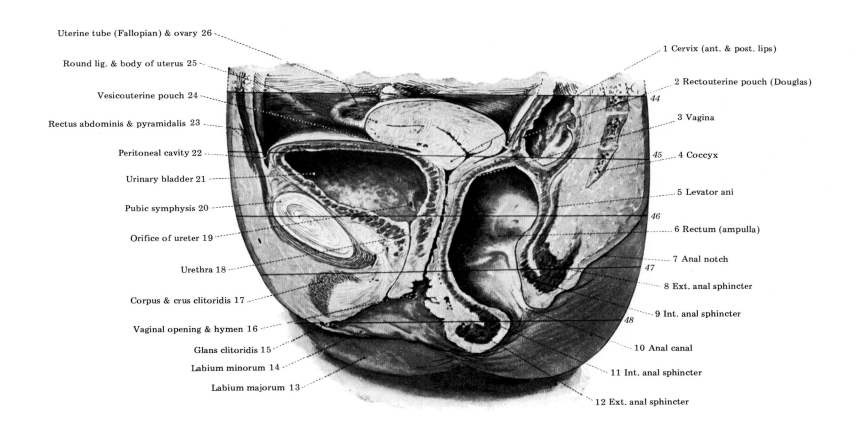

Uterine tube (Fallopian) & ovary 26

Round lig. & body of uterus 25

Vesicouterine pouch 24

Rectus abdominis & pyramidalis 23

Peritoneal cavity 22

Urinary bladder 21

Pubic symphysis 20

Orifice of ureter 19

Urethra 18

Corpus & crus clitoridis 17

Vaginal opening & hymen 16

Glans clitoridis 15

Labium minorum 14

Labium majorum 13

1 Cervix (ant. & post. lips)

2 Rectouterine pouch (Douglas)

44

3 Vagina

45   4 Coccyx

5 Levator ani

46

6 Rectum (ampulla)

7 Anal notch

47

8 Ext. anal sphincter

9 Int. anal sphincter

48

10 Anal canal

11 Int. anal sphincter

12 Ext. anal sphincter

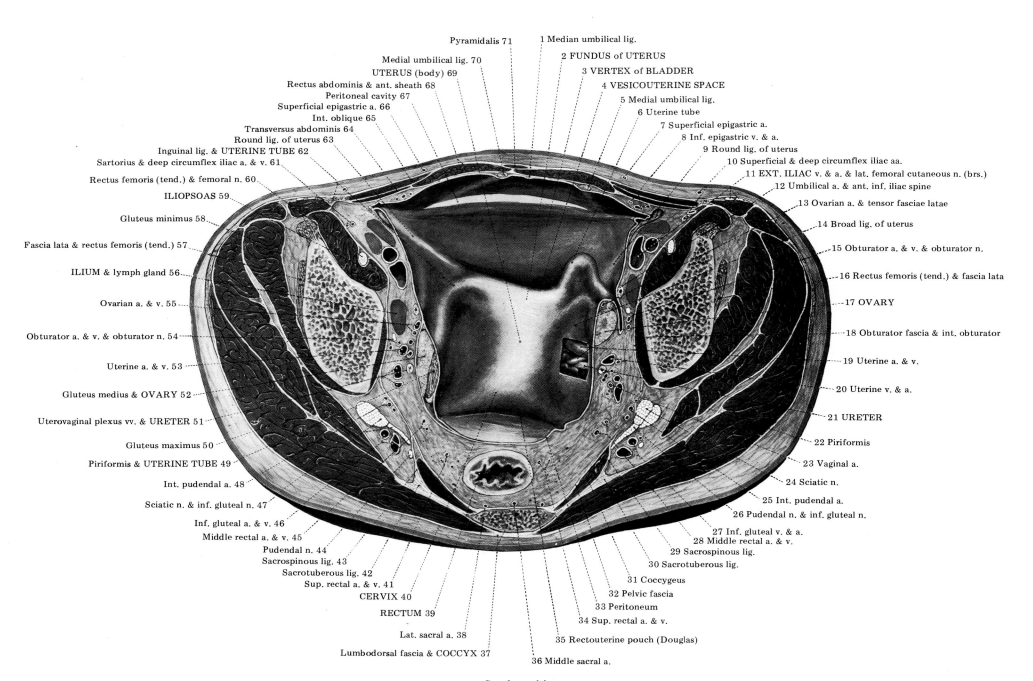

Pyramidalis 71
1 Median umbilical lig.
Medial umbilical lig. 70
2 FUNDUS of UTERUS
UTERUS (body) 69
3 VERTEX of BLADDER
Rectus abdominis & ant. sheath 68
4 VESICOUTERINE SPACE
Peritoneal cavity 67
5 Medial umbilical lig.
Superficial epigastric a. 66
6 Uterine tube
Int. oblique 65
7 Superficial epigastric a.
Transversus abdominis 64
8 Inf. epigastric v. & a.
Round lig. of uterus 63
9 Round lig. of uterus
Inguinal lig. & UTERINE TUBE 62
10 Superficial & deep circumflex iliac aa.
Sartorius & deep circumflex iliac a. & v. 61
11 EXT. ILIAC v. & a. & lat. femoral cutaneous n. (brs.)
Rectus femoris (tend.) & femoral n. 60
12 Umbilical a. & ant. inf. iliac spine
ILIOPSOAS 59
13 Ovarian a. & tensor fasciae latae
Gluteus minimus 58
14 Broad lig. of uterus
Fascia lata & rectus femoris (tend.) 57
15 Obturator a. & v. & obturator n.
ILIUM & lymph gland 56
16 Rectus femoris (tend.) & fascia lata
Ovarian a. & v. 55
17 OVARY
Obturator a. & v. & obturator n. 54
18 Obturator fascia & int. obturator
Uterine a. & v. 53
19 Uterine a. & v.
Gluteus medius & OVARY 52
20 Uterine v. & a.
Uterovaginal plexus vv. & URETER 51
21 URETER
Gluteus maximus 50
22 Piriformis
Piriformis & UTERINE TUBE 49
23 Vaginal a.
Int. pudendal a. 48
24 Sciatic n.
Sciatic n. & inf. gluteal n. 47
25 Int. pudendal a.
Inf. gluteal a. & v. 46
26 Pudendal n. & inf. gluteal n.
Middle rectal a. & v. 45
27 Inf. gluteal v. & a.
Pudendal n. 44
28 Middle rectal a. & v.
Sacrospinous lig. 43
29 Sacrospinous lig.
Sacrotuberous lig. 42
30 Sacrotuberous lig.
Sup. rectal a. & v. 41
31 Coccygeus
CERVIX 40
32 Pelvic fascia
RECTUM 39
33 Peritoneum
34 Sup. rectal a. & v.
Lat. sacral a. 38
35 Rectouterine pouch (Douglas)
Lumbodorsal fascia & COCCYX 37
36 Middle sacral a.

Section 44

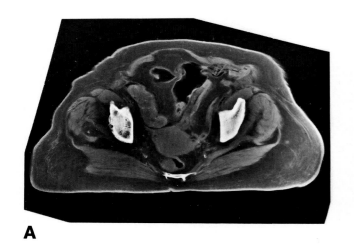

A

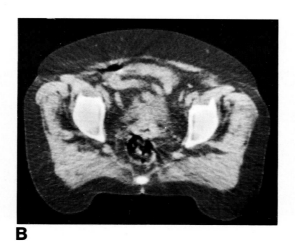

B

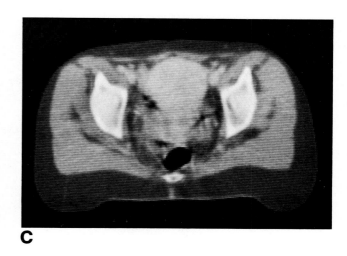

C

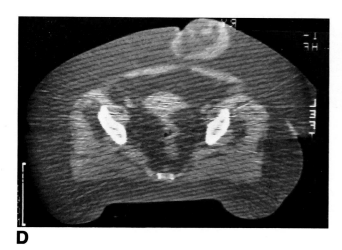

D

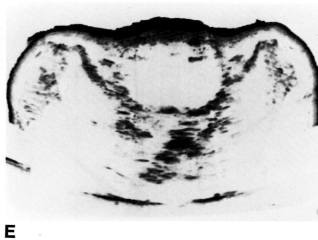

E

SECTION 44

Figure (**A**) is an x-ray of cross-section taken through a cadaver; (**B**), (**C**), and (**D**) are CT scans of patients. The cervix (40) and part of the uterus (69) are seen at the level of the roof of the acetabulum (56). The ovary (17) can be seen occasionally (**D**), but may be difficult to identify. The bladder (3) lies anteriorly and the rectum (39) posteriorly. The iliac vessels (11) are medial to the iliopsoas muscle (59). The coccyx (37) is also evident posteriorly. The abdominal rectus muscles (68) can be seen anteriorly.

In the echogram (**E**), the bladder (3) is distended with urine to permit better visualization of the pelvic structures. The adnexal structures can be seen just lateral to the bladder and medial to the iliac bone. The fundus of the uterus (69) is poorly defined just posterior to the bladder, and slightly to the right side.

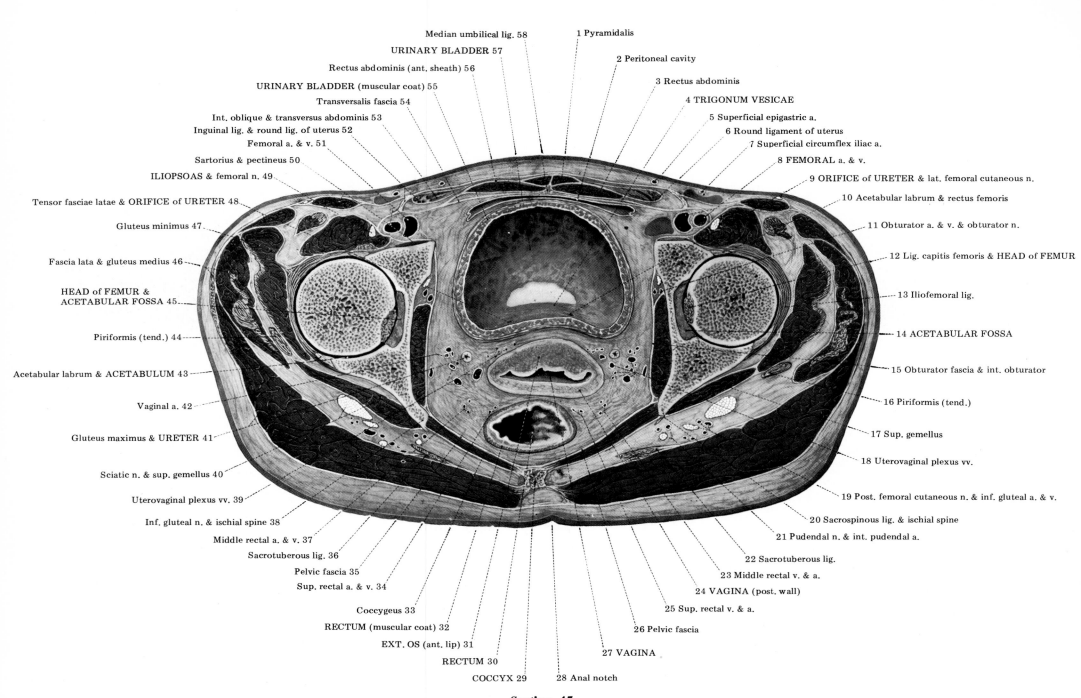

Median umbilical lig. 58
URINARY BLADDER 57
Rectus abdominis (ant. sheath) 56
URINARY BLADDER (muscular coat) 55
Transversalis fascia 54
Int. oblique & transversus abdominis 53
Inguinal lig. & round lig. of uterus 52
Femoral a. & v. 51
Sartorius & pectineus 50
ILIOPSOAS & femoral n. 49
Tensor fasciae latae & ORIFICE of URETER 48
Gluteus minimus 47
Fascia lata & gluteus medius 46
HEAD of FEMUR &
ACETABULAR FOSSA 45
Piriformis (tend.) 44
Acetabular labrum & ACETABULUM 43
Vaginal a. 42
Gluteus maximus & URETER 41
Sciatic n. & sup. gemellus 40
Uterovaginal plexus vv. 39
Inf. gluteal n. & ischial spine 38
Middle rectal a. & v. 37
Sacrotuberous lig. 36
Pelvic fascia 35
Sup. rectal a. & v. 34
Coccygeus 33
RECTUM (muscular coat) 32
EXT. OS (ant. lip) 31
RECTUM 30
COCCYX 29
28 Anal notch

1 Pyramidalis
2 Peritoneal cavity
3 Rectus abdominis
4 TRIGONUM VESICAE
5 Superficial epigastric a.
6 Round ligament of uterus
7 Superficial circumflex iliac a.
8 FEMORAL a. & v.
9 ORIFICE of URETER & lat. femoral cutaneous n.
10 Acetabular labrum & rectus femoris
11 Obturator a. & v. & obturator n.
12 Lig. capitis femoris & HEAD of FEMUR
13 Iliofemoral lig.
14 ACETABULAR FOSSA
15 Obturator fascia & int. obturator
16 Piriformis (tend.)
17 Sup. gemellus
18 Uterovaginal plexus vv.
19 Post. femoral cutaneous n. & inf. gluteal a. & v.
20 Sacrospinous lig. & ischial spine
21 Pudendal n. & int. pudendal a.
22 Sacrotuberous lig.
23 Middle rectal v. & a.
24 VAGINA (post. wall)
25 Sup. rectal v. & a.
26 Pelvic fascia
27 VAGINA

Section 45

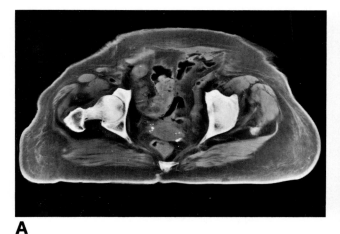

A

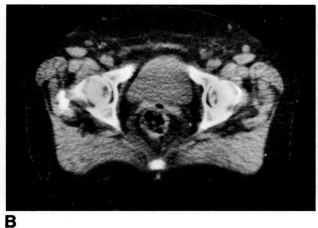

B

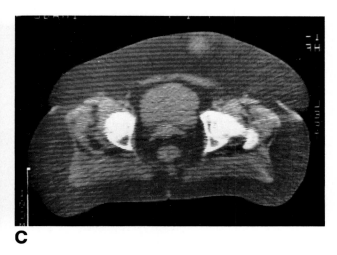

C

SECTION 45

Figure (**A**) is an x-ray of a transverse section from a female cadaver; (**B**), (**C**), and (**D**) are CT scans of female patients. All sections were taken at the level of the acetabulum. Note the femoral head with the notch for the ligamentum teres (12, 45), the ischial spine (20), and the coccyx (29) with the coccygeus muscle (33). The femoral vessels (8) are medial to the iliopsoas muscle (49). The vagina (**B**-31) and surrounding utero-vaginal plexus can be seen lying between the bladder (**B**-57) and the rectum (**B**-30). Note the calcifications in the utero-vaginal plexus in the cadaver (**A**-18).

In the echogram (**E**), the bladder (57) is again well distended. The body of the uterus is now clearly identified just posterior to the bladder and slightly to the right. Some fainter echoes arising from the rectum are seen somewhat to the left of the uterus. Anteriorly, the iliopsoas muscles (49) can be seen in front of the acetabulum. Since the ultrasonic visualization of the lower sections of the female pelvis do not differ significantly from those of the male pelvis shown in Sections 41 to 43, ultrasonic views of these areas are not included in this atlas.

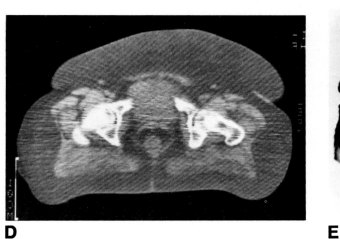

D

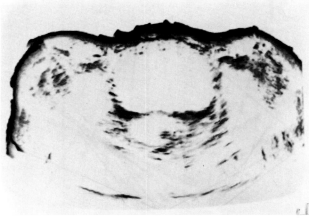

E

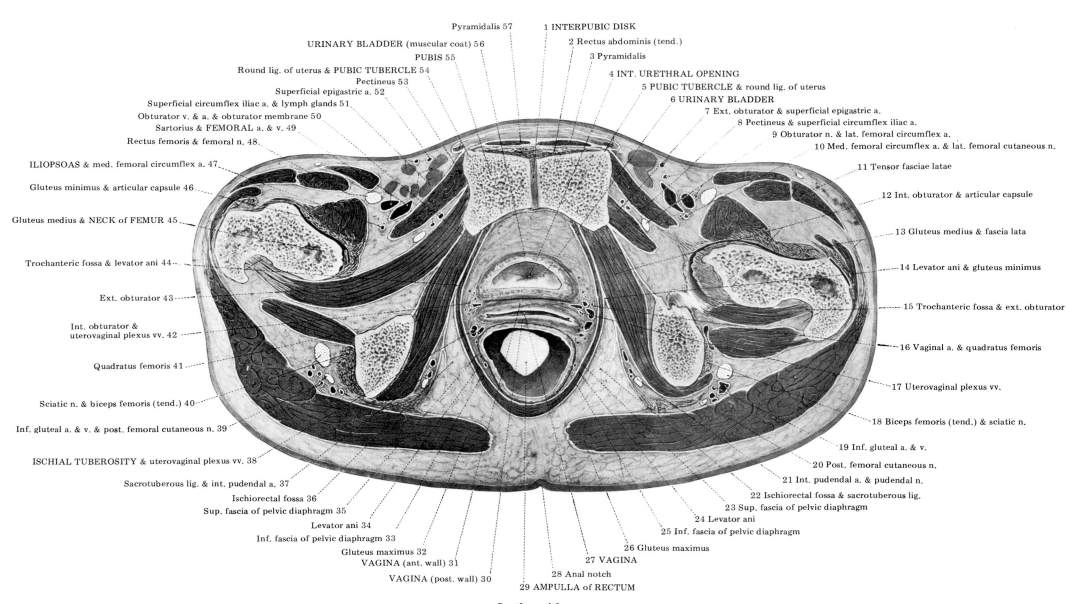

Pyramidalis 57

URINARY BLADDER (muscular coat) 56

PUBIS 55

Round lig. of uterus & PUBIC TUBERCLE 54

Pectineus 53

Superficial epigastric a. 52

Superficial circumflex iliac a. & lymph glands 51

Obturator v. & a. & obturator membrane 50

Sartorius & FEMORAL a. & v. 49

Rectus femoris & femoral n. 48

ILIOPSOAS & med. femoral circumflex a. 47

Gluteus minimus & articular capsule 46

Gluteus medius & NECK of FEMUR 45

Trochanteric fossa & levator ani 44

Ext. obturator 43

Int. obturator &
uterovaginal plexus vv. 42

Quadratus femoris 41

Sciatic n. & biceps femoris (tend.) 40

Inf. gluteal a. & v. & post. femoral cutaneous n. 39

ISCHIAL TUBEROSITY & uterovaginal plexus vv. 38

Sacrotuberous lig. & int. pudendal a. 37

Ischiorectal fossa 36

Sup. fascia of pelvic diaphragm 35

Levator ani 34

Inf. fascia of pelvic diaphragm 33

Gluteus maximus 32

VAGINA (ant. wall) 31

VAGINA (post. wall) 30

1 INTERPUBIC DISK

2 Rectus abdominis (tend.)

3 Pyramidalis

4 INT. URETHRAL OPENING

5 PUBIC TUBERCLE & round lig. of uterus

6 URINARY BLADDER

7 Ext. obturator & superficial epigastric a.

8 Pectineus & superficial circumflex iliac a.

9 Obturator n. & lat. femoral circumflex a.

10 Med. femoral circumflex a. & lat. femoral cutaneous n.

11 Tensor fasciae latae

12 Int. obturator & articular capsule

13 Gluteus medius & fascia lata

14 Levator ani & gluteus minimus

15 Trochanteric fossa & ext. obturator

16 Vaginal a. & quadratus femoris

17 Uterovaginal plexus vv.

18 Biceps femoris (tend.) & sciatic n.

19 Inf. gluteal a. & v.

20 Post. femoral cutaneous n.

21 Int. pudendal a. & pudendal n.

22 Ischiorectal fossa & sacrotuberous lig.

23 Sup. fascia of pelvic diaphragm

24 Levator ani

25 Inf. fascia of pelvic diaphragm

26 Gluteus maximus

27 VAGINA

28 Anal notch

29 AMPULLA of RECTUM

Section 46

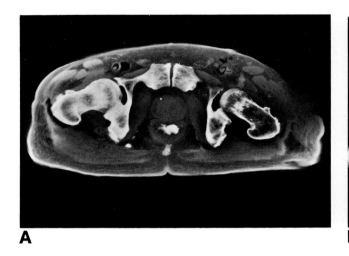

A

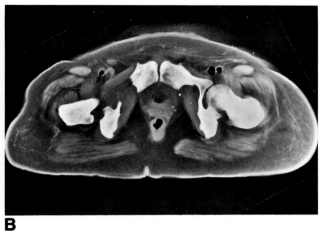

B

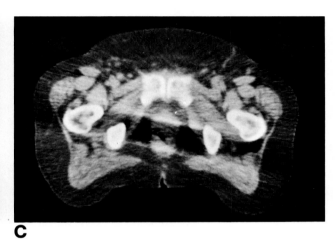

C

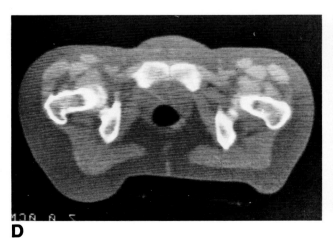

D

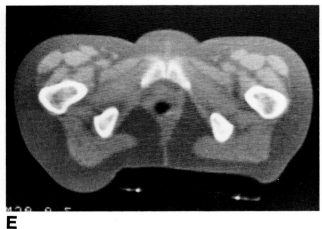

E

SECTION 46

Figures (**A**) and (**B**) are x-rays of cross sections of cadavers, whereas (**C**), (**D**), and (**E**) are CT scans of patients taken at similar levels. All show the symphysis pubis (1), and the ischial tuberosity (38) with the internal obturator muscles (12) in between. The vagina (27) does not contain air and is thus hard to distinguish from the floor of the bladder (56) and the rectum (29). The levator ani (24) surrounds these structures and separates them from the ischio-rectal fossa (22). Also note the external obturator muscle (43) originating from the pubis (55) and inserting on the femoral neck (45). The femoral vessels (49) and nodes are anteromedial to the iliopsoas (47). The gluteus maximus (26) and subcutaneous fat are distorted by the position of the patient.

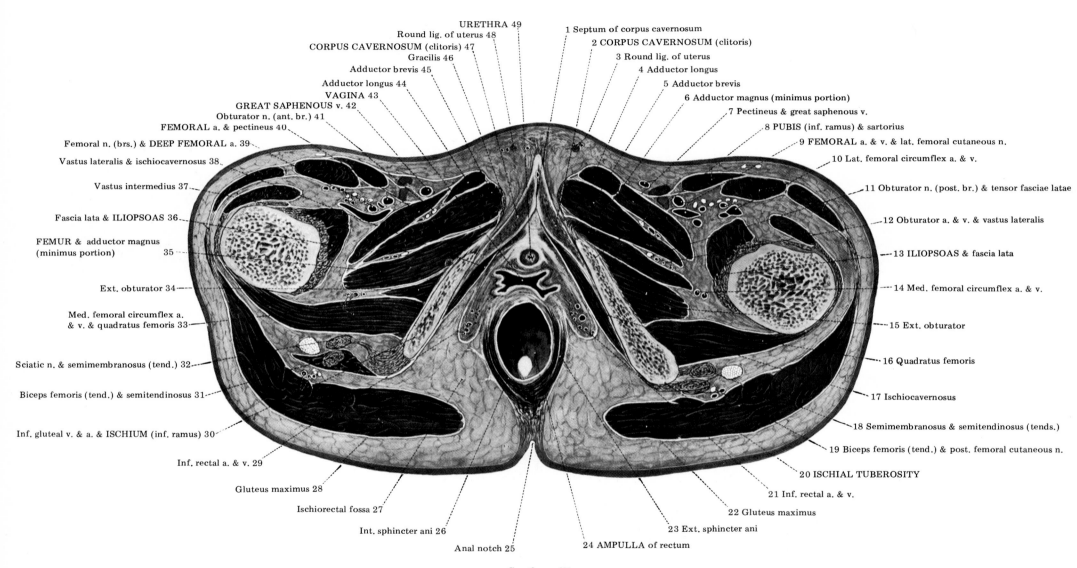

URETHRA 49
Round lig. of uterus 48
CORPUS CAVERNOSUM (clitoris) 47
Gracilis 46
Adductor brevis 45
Adductor longus 44
VAGINA 43
GREAT SAPHENOUS v. 42
Obturator n. (ant. br.) 41
FEMORAL a. & pectineus 40
Femoral n. (brs.) & DEEP FEMORAL a. 39
Vastus lateralis & ischiocavernosus 38
Vastus intermedius 37
Fascia lata & ILIOPSOAS 36
FEMUR & adductor magnus
(minimus portion)   35
Ext. obturator 34
Med. femoral circumflex a.
& v. & quadratus femoris 33
Sciatic n. & semimembranosus (tend.) 32
Biceps femoris (tend.) & semitendinosus 31
Inf. gluteal v. & a. & ISCHIUM (inf. ramus) 30
Inf. rectal a. & v. 29
Gluteus maximus 28
Ischiorectal fossa 27
Int. sphincter ani 26
Anal notch 25

1 Septum of corpus cavernosum
2 CORPUS CAVERNOSUM (clitoris)
3 Round lig. of uterus
4 Adductor longus
5 Adductor brevis
6 Adductor magnus (minimus portion)
7 Pectineus & great saphenous v.
8 PUBIS (inf. ramus) & sartorius
9 FEMORAL a. & v. & lat. femoral cutaneous n.
10 Lat. femoral circumflex a. & v.
11 Obturator n. (post. br.) & tensor fasciae latae
12 Obturator a. & v. & vastus lateralis
13 ILIOPSOAS & fascia lata
14 Med. femoral circumflex a. & v.
15 Ext. obturator
16 Quadratus femoris
17 Ischiocavernosus
18 Semimembranosus & semitendinosus (tends.)
19 Biceps femoris (tend.) & post. femoral cutaneous n.
20 ISCHIAL TUBEROSITY
21 Inf. rectal a. & v.
22 Gluteus maximus
23 Ext. sphincter ani
24 AMPULLA of rectum

Section 47

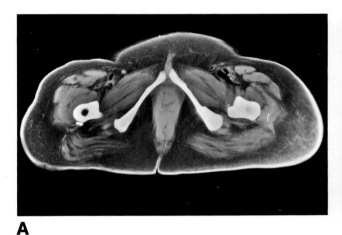

A

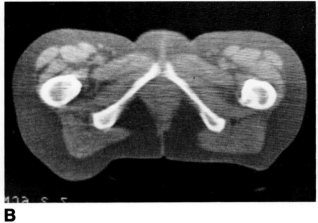

B

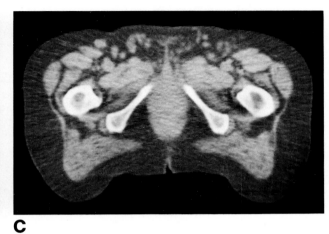

C

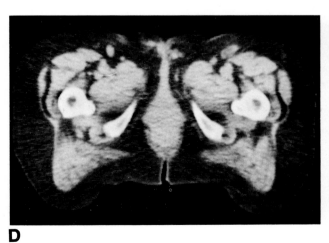

D

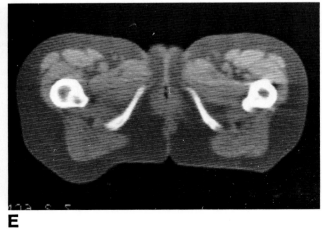

E

SECTION 47

An x-ray of a specimen (**A**) and CT scans of four different patients (**B**), (**C**), (**D**), and (**E**) were taken at the level of the inferior border of the symphysis (8) and ischial tuberosity (20). They show the region of the urethra (49), vagina (43), and anus (24), which are usually difficult to distinguish because of the lack of air. The corpus cavernosum of the clitoris (2) can be seen anteriorly. Note the femoral vessels (40) and nodes anteromedial to the iliopsoas muscle (36). Both femurs (35) are seen in cross section.

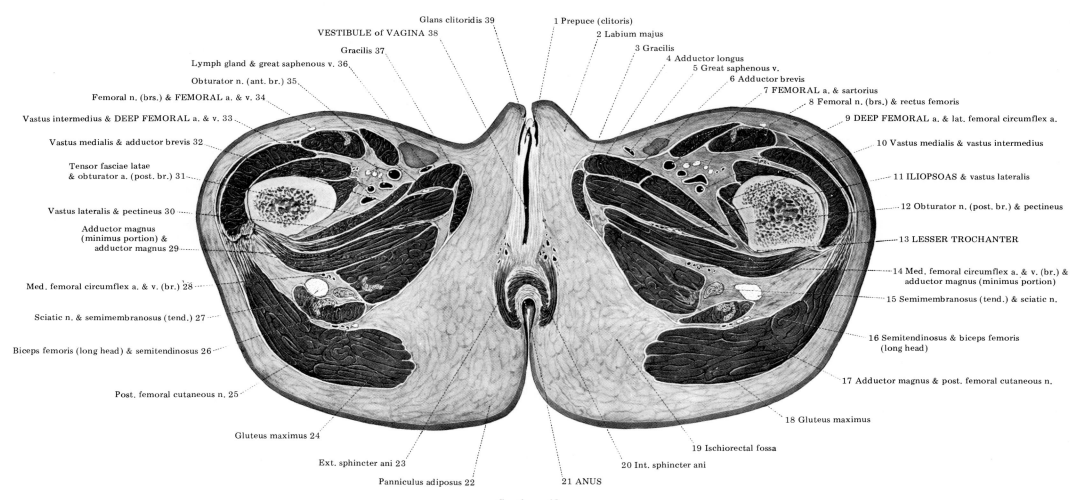

Glans clitoridis 39

VESTIBULE of VAGINA 38

Gracilis 37

Lymph gland & great saphenous v. 36

Obturator n. (ant. br.) 35

Femoral n. (brs.) & FEMORAL a. & v. 34

Vastus intermedius & DEEP FEMORAL a. & v. 33

Vastus medialis & adductor brevis 32

Tensor fasciae latae
& obturator a. (post. br.) 31

Vastus lateralis & pectineus 30

Adductor magnus
(minimus portion) &
adductor magnus 29

Med. femoral circumflex a. & v. (br.) 28

Sciatic n. & semimembranosus (tend.) 27

Biceps femoris (long head) & semitendinosus 26

Post. femoral cutaneous n. 25

Gluteus maximus 24

Ext. sphincter ani 23

Panniculus adiposus 22

1 Prepuce (clitoris)

2 Labium majus

3 Gracilis

4 Adductor longus

5 Great saphenous v.

6 Adductor brevis

7 FEMORAL a. & sartorius

8 Femoral n. (brs.) & rectus femoris

9 DEEP FEMORAL a. & lat. femoral circumflex a.

10 Vastus medialis & vastus intermedius

11 ILIOPSOAS & vastus lateralis

12 Obturator n. (post. br.) & pectineus

13 LESSER TROCHANTER

14 Med. femoral circumflex a. & v. (br.) &
adductor magnus (minimus portion)

15 Semimembranosus (tend.) & sciatic n.

16 Semitendinosus & biceps femoris
(long head)

17 Adductor magnus & post. femoral cutaneous n.

18 Gluteus maximus

19 Ischiorectal fossa

20 Int. sphincter ani

21 ANUS

Section 48

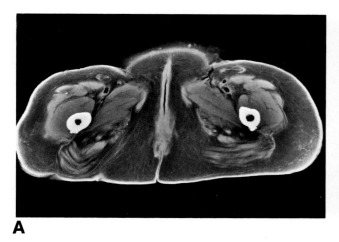

A

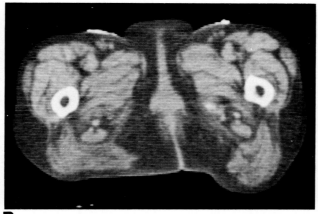

B

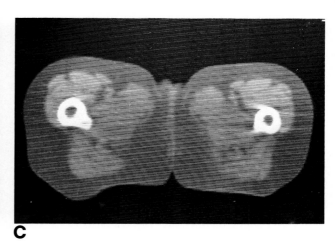

C

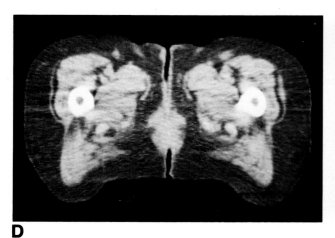

D

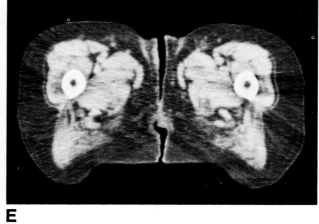

E

SECTION 48

An x-ray of a specimen (**A**) and four CT scans (**B**), (**C**), (**D**), (**E**) at slightly different levels show the clitoris (1), labium majus (2), vestibule of the vagina (38), and the anus (21). The femoral vessels (7) can be identified anteromedial to the femur (13) on these sections taken close to the region of the lesser trochanter (13), which is the site of insertion for the iliopsoas (11). Barium paste has been used on the skin (**B**) as a marker.

KEY FIGURES X AND XI   These key figures represent a frontal view of the left arm. The bones, the principal arteries, veins, nerves, and muscles are shown. The levels of the following sections with reference to the various structures are indicated by the transverse lines 49–63.

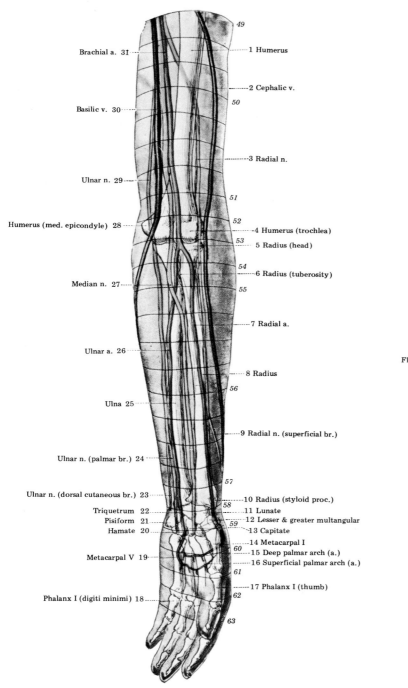

Brachial a. 31

1 Humerus

2 Cephalic v.

Basilic v. 30

3 Radial n.

Ulnar n. 29

Humerus (med. epicondyle) 28

4 Humerus (trochlea)

5 Radius (head)

6 Radius (tuberosity)

Median n. 27

7 Radial a.

Ulnar a. 26

8 Radius

Ulna 25

9 Radial n. (superficial br.)

Ulnar n. (palmar br.) 24

Ulnar n. (dorsal cutaneous br.) 23

10 Radius (styloid proc.)

Triquetrum 22

11 Lunate

Pisiform 21

12 Lesser & greater multangular

Hamate 20

13 Capitate

14 Metacarpal I

15 Deep palmar arch (a.)

Metacarpal V 19

16 Superficial palmar arch (a.)

17 Phalanx I (thumb)

Phalanx I (digiti minimi) 18

KEY FIGURE X

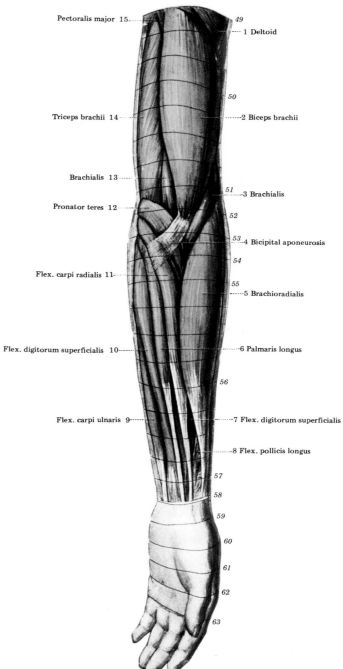

Pectoralis major 15

1 Deltoid

Triceps brachii 14

2 Biceps brachii

Brachialis 13

3 Brachialis

Pronator teres 12

4 Bicipital aponeurosis

Flex. carpi radialis 11

5 Brachioradialis

Flex. digitorum superficialis 10

6 Palmaris longus

Flex. carpi ulnaris 9

7 Flex. digitorum superficialis

8 Flex. pollicis longus

KEY FIGURE XI

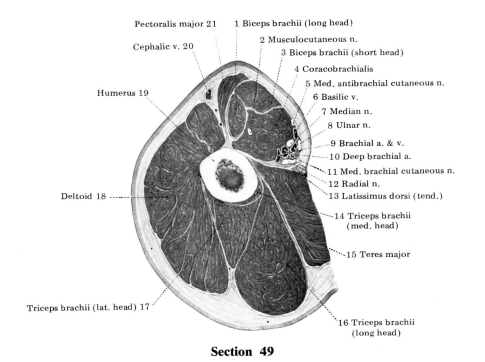

Pectoralis major 21   1 Biceps brachii (long head)

Cephalic v. 20

    2 Musculocutaneous n.

    3 Biceps brachii (short head)

    4 Coracobrachialis

Humerus 19

    5 Med. antibrachial cutaneous n.

    6 Basilic v.

    7 Median n.

    8 Ulnar n.

    9 Brachial a. & v.

    10 Deep brachial a.

    11 Med. brachial cutaneous n.

    12 Radial n.

    13 Latissimus dorsi (tend.)

Deltoid 18

    14 Triceps brachii (med. head)

    15 Teres major

Triceps brachii (lat. head) 17

    16 Triceps brachii (long head)

Section 49

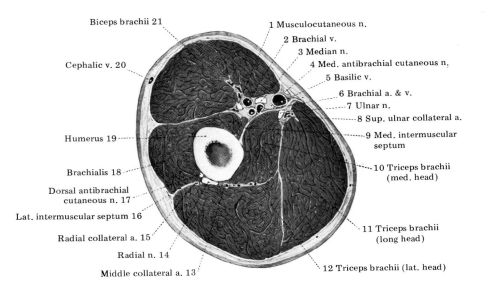

Biceps brachii 21   1 Musculocutaneous n.

    2 Brachial v.

    3 Median n.

Cephalic v. 20

    4 Med. antibrachial cutaneous n.

    5 Basilic v.

    6 Brachial a. & v.

    7 Ulnar n.

    8 Sup. ulnar collateral a.

    9 Med. intermuscular septum

Humerus 19

Brachialis 18

    10 Triceps brachii (med. head)

Dorsal antibrachial cutaneous n. 17

Lat. intermuscular septum 16

    11 Triceps brachii (long head)

Radial collateral a. 15

Radial n. 14

Middle collateral a. 13   12 Triceps brachii (lat. head)

Section 50

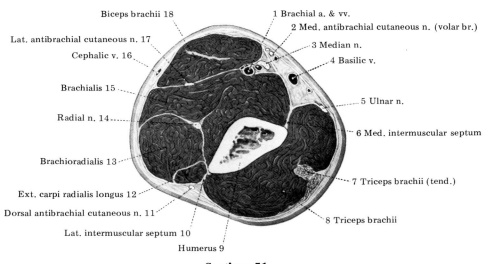

Biceps brachii 18   1 Brachial a. & vv.

    2 Med. antibrachial cutaneous n. (volar br.)

Lat. antibrachial cutaneous n. 17

    3 Median n.

Cephalic v. 16

    4 Basilic v.

Brachialis 15

    5 Ulnar n.

Radial n. 14

    6 Med. intermuscular septum

Brachioradialis 13

    7 Triceps brachii (tend.)

Ext. carpi radialis longus 12

Dorsal antibrachial cutaneous n. 11

    8 Triceps brachii

Lat. intermuscular septum 10

Humerus 9

Section 51

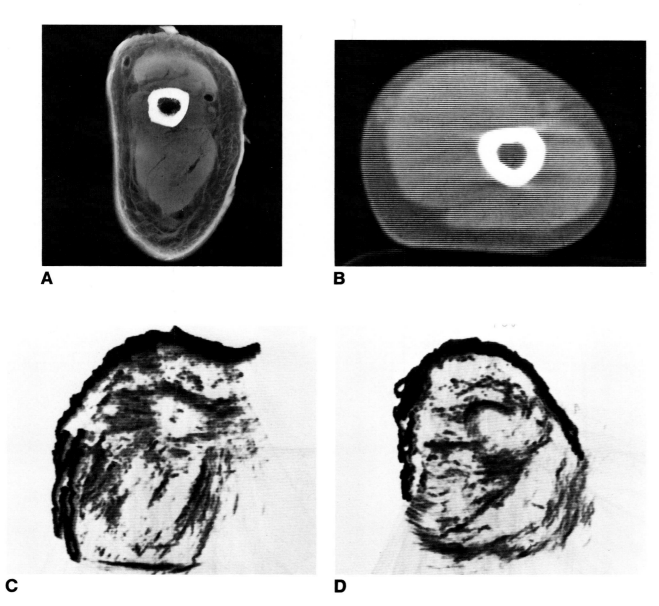

A

B

C

D

SECTIONS 49, 50, 51

X-ray of a specimen (**A**), CT scan (**B**), and ultrasound (**C**) and (**D**) are taken through the proximal humerus. Major muscle bundles can be identified: the biceps anterolaterally, the brachial muscle laterally, and the triceps posteromedially. The basilic and cephalic veins are easily seen because of their subcutaneous position which contains more fat.

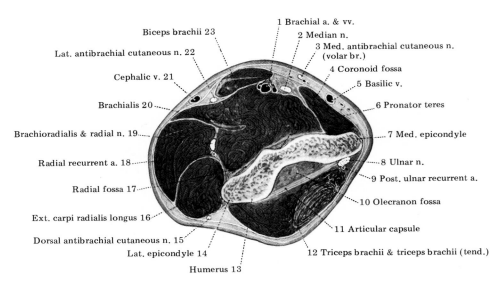

Biceps brachii 23

Lat. antibrachial cutaneous n. 22

Cephalic v. 21

Brachialis 20

Brachioradialis & radial n. 19

Radial recurrent a. 18

Radial fossa 17

Ext. carpi radialis longus 16

Dorsal antibrachial cutaneous n. 15

Lat. epicondyle 14

Humerus 13

1 Brachial a. & vv.
2 Median n.
3 Med. antibrachial cutaneous n. (volar br.)
4 Coronoid fossa
5 Basilic v.
6 Pronator teres
7 Med. epicondyle
8 Ulnar n.
9 Post. ulnar recurrent a.
10 Olecranon fossa
11 Articular capsule
12 Triceps brachii & triceps brachii (tend.)

Section 52

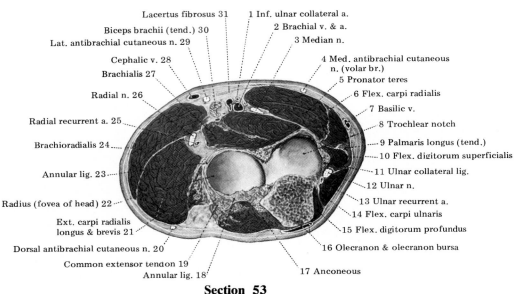

Lacertus fibrosus 31
Biceps brachii (tend.) 30
Lat. antibrachial cutaneous n. 29
Cephalic v. 28
Brachialis 27
Radial n. 26
Radial recurrent a. 25
Brachioradialis 24
Annular lig. 23
Radius (fovea of head) 22
Ext. carpi radialis longus & brevis 21
Dorsal antibrachial cutaneous n. 20
Common extensor tendon 19
Annular lig. 18

1 Inf. ulnar collateral a.
2 Brachial v. & a.
3 Median n.
4 Med. antibrachial cutaneous n. (volar br.)
5 Pronator teres
6 Flex. carpi radialis
7 Basilic v.
8 Trochlear notch
9 Palmaris longus (tend.)
10 Flex. digitorum superficialis
11 Ulnar collateral lig.
12 Ulnar n.
13 Ulnar recurrent a.
14 Flex. carpi ulnaris
15 Flex. digitorum profundus
16 Olecranon & olecranon bursa
17 Anconeous

Section 53

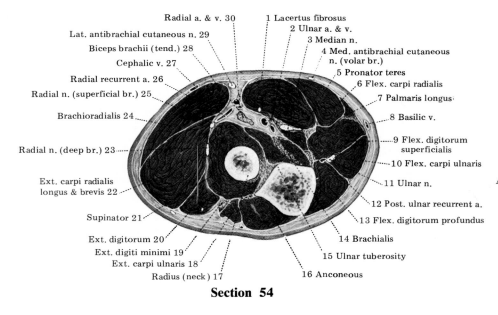

Radial a. & v. 30
Lat. antibrachial cutaneous n. 29
Biceps brachii (tend.) 28
Cephalic v. 27
Radial recurrent a. 26
Radial n. (superficial br.) 25
Brachioradialis 24
Radial n. (deep br.) 23
Ext. carpi radialis longus & brevis 22
Supinator 21
Ext. digitorum 20
Ext. digiti minimi 19
Ext. carpi ulnaris 18
Radius (neck) 17

1 Lacertus fibrosus
2 Ulnar a. & v.
3 Median n.
4 Med. antibrachial cutaneous n. (volar br.)
5 Pronator teres
6 Flex. carpi radialis
7 Palmaris longus
8 Basilic v.
9 Flex. digitorum superficialis
10 Flex. carpi ulnaris
11 Ulnar n.
12 Post. ulnar recurrent a.
13 Flex. digitorum profundus
14 Brachialis
15 Ulnar tuberosity
16 Anconeous

Section 54

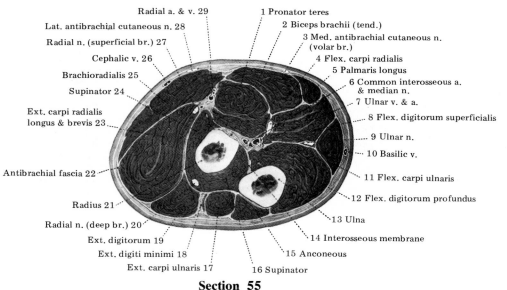

Radial a. & v. 29
Lat. antibrachial cutaneous n. 28
Radial n. (superficial br.) 27
Cephalic v. 26
Brachioradialis 25
Supinator 24
Ext. carpi radialis longus & brevis 23
Antibrachial fascia 22
Radius 21
Radial n. (deep br.) 20
Ext. digitorum 19
Ext. digiti minimi 18
Ext. carpi ulnaris 17

1 Pronator teres
2 Biceps brachii (tend.)
3 Med. antibrachial cutaneous n. (volar br.)
4 Flex. carpi radialis
5 Palmaris longus
6 Common interosseous a. & median n.
7 Ulnar v. & a.
8 Flex. digitorum superficialis
9 Ulnar n.
10 Basilic v.
11 Flex. carpi ulnaris
12 Flex. digitorum profundus
13 Ulna
14 Interosseous membrane
15 Anconeous
16 Supinator

Section 55

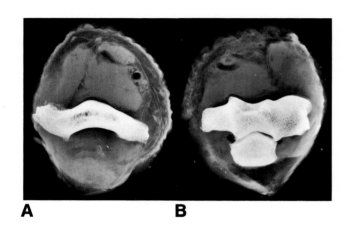

A   **B**

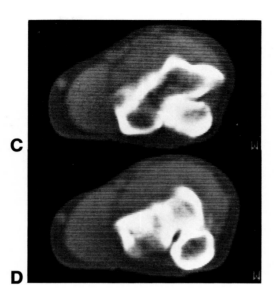

C

D

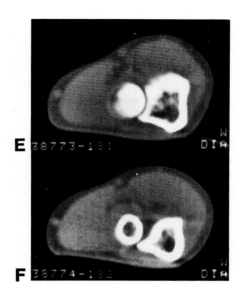

E

F

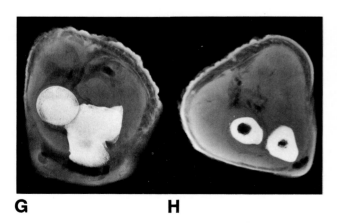

G   **H**

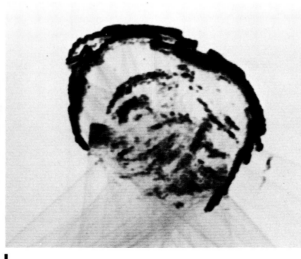

I

SECTIONS 52, 53, 54, 55

X-ray specimens (**A**) (**B**), (**G**), and (**H**) and CT scans (**C**), (**D**),(**E**), and (**F**) through the elbow show in sequence the olecranon fossa with the medial and lateral epicondyles (**A**); the olecranon process (**B**), (**C**), and (**D**); the head of the radius articulating with the ulna (**E**), (**F**), and (**G**); and the proximal forearm (**H**). The cephalic and basilic veins are the easiest of the vascular structures to identify since they are surrounded by subcutaneous fat. The ulnar artery and vein can also been seen (**E**), (**F**), and (**H**) immediately anterior to the bones, whereas the radial artery and vein are more superficial in location. Note the supinator muscle surrounding the radius (**E**), (**F**), (**G**), and (**H**) which is also evident by ultrasound (**I**). The large muscle mass of the brachioradials and extensor carpi radialis are seen laterally (**H**) and (**I**) and the flexor muscles anteromedially (**H**) and (**I**).

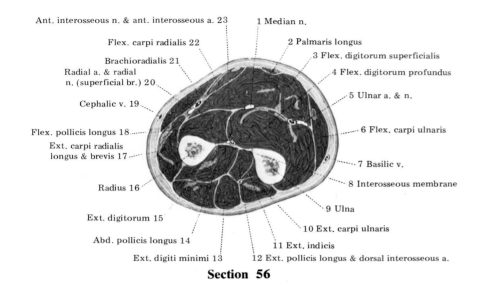

Ant. interosseous n. & ant. interosseous a. 23
Flex. carpi radialis 22
Brachioradialis 21
Radial a. & radial
n. (superficial br.) 20
Cephalic v. 19
Flex. pollicis longus 18
Ext. carpi radialis
longus & brevis 17
Radius 16
Ext. digitorum 15
Abd. pollicis longus 14
Ext. digiti minimi 13

1 Median n.
2 Palmaris longus
3 Flex. digitorum superficialis
4 Flex. digitorum profundus
5 Ulnar a. & n.
6 Flex. carpi ulnaris
7 Basilic v.
8 Interosseous membrane
9 Ulna
10 Ext. carpi ulnaris
11 Ext. indicis
12 Ext. pollicis longus & dorsal interosseous a.

Section 56

Palmaris longus (tend.) 25
Median n. 24
Flex. carpi radialis (tend.) 23
Flex. pollicis longus 22
Radial a. 21
Radius 20
Radial n. (superficial br.) 19
Brachioradialis (tend.) 18
Abd. pollicis longus 17
Ext. pollicis brevis (tend.) 16
Radial n. (superficial br.) 15
Ext. carpi radialis
longus & brevis (tend.) 14
Ext. pollicis longus (tend.) 13
Ext. digitorum (tend.) 12
Ext. indicis 11

1 Flex. digitorum superficialis
2 Flex. digitorum profundus
3 Ulnar a. & ulnar n.
(palmar cutaneous br.)
4 Flex. carpi ulnaris
5 Basilic v.
6 Ulnar n. (dorsal br.)
7 Pronator quadratus
8 Ulna
9 Ext. carpi ulnaris (tend.)
10 Ext. digiti minimi (tend.)

Section 57

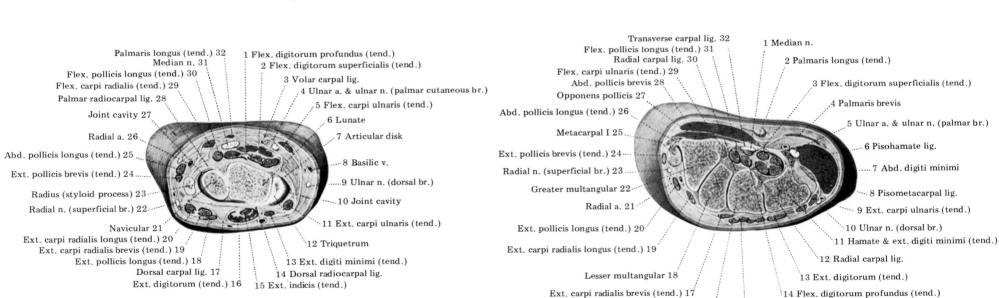

Palmaris longus (tend.) 32
Median n. 31
Flex. pollicis longus (tend.) 30
Flex. carpi radialis (tend.) 29
Palmar radiocarpal lig. 28
Joint cavity 27
Radial a. 26
Abd. pollicis longus (tend.) 25
Ext. pollicis brevis (tend.) 24
Radius (styloid process) 23
Radial n. (superficial br.) 22
Navicular 21
Ext. carpi radialis longus (tend.) 20
Ext. carpi radialis brevis (tend.) 19
Ext. pollicis longus (tend.) 18
Dorsal carpal lig. 17
Ext. digitorum (tend.) 16

1 Flex. digitorum profundus (tend.)
2 Flex. digitorum superficialis (tend.)
3 Volar carpal lig.
4 Ulnar a. & ulnar n. (palmar cutaneous br.)
5 Flex. carpi ulnaris (tend.)
6 Lunate
7 Articular disk
8 Basilic v.
9 Ulnar n. (dorsal br.)
10 Joint cavity
11 Ext. carpi ulnaris (tend.)
12 Triquetrum
13 Ext. digiti minimi (tend.)
14 Dorsal radiocarpal lig.
15 Ext. indicis (tend.)

Section 58

Transverse carpal lig. 32
Flex. pollicis longus (tend.) 31
Radial carpal lig. 30
Flex. carpi ulnaris (tend.) 29
Abd. pollicis brevis 28
Opponens pollicis 27
Abd. pollicis longus (tend.) 26
Metacarpal I 25
Ext. pollicis brevis (tend.) 24
Radial n. (superficial br.) 23
Greater multangular 22
Radial a. 21
Ext. pollicis longus (tend.) 20
Ext. carpi radialis longus (tend.) 19
Lesser multangular 18
Ext. carpi radialis brevis (tend.) 17
Capitate 16

1 Median n.
2 Palmaris longus (tend.)
3 Flex. digitorum superficialis (tend.)
4 Palmaris brevis
5 Ulnar a. & ulnar n. (palmar br.)
6 Pisohamate lig.
7 Abd. digiti minimi
8 Pisometacarpal lig.
9 Ext. carpi ulnaris (tend.)
10 Ulnar n. (dorsal br.)
11 Hamate & ext. digiti minimi (tend.)
12 Radial carpal lig.
13 Ext. digitorum (tend.)
14 Flex. digitorum profundus (tend.)
15 Ext. indicis (tend.)

Section 59

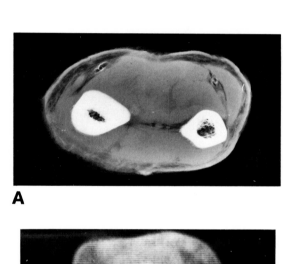

A

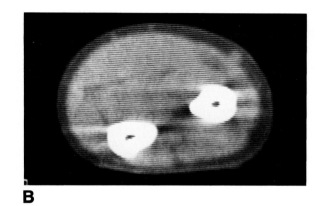

B

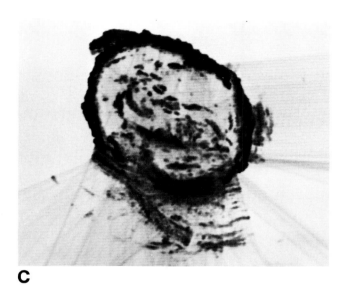

C

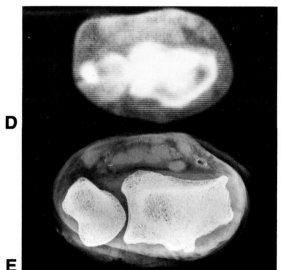

D

E

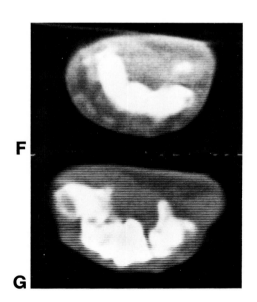

F

G

SECTIONS 56, 57, 58, 59

The radius, ulna, and interosseous membrane are evident on the x-ray of the specimen (**A**), CT scan (**B**), and ultrasound (**C**). The flexor muscles lie anteriorly, the extensor muscles posteriorly; the basiliac and cephalic veins are easier to see in their more subcutaneous position than the ulnar artery, which is deep to the flexor carpi ulnaris. The radial artery lies between the flexor carpi radialis and flexor pollicis longus.

A CT scan (**D**) and x-ray of a specimen (**E**) are taken through the articulation of the radius and ulna; scans (**F**) and (**G**) through the carpal bones clearly show the carpal tunnel containing the flexor tendons.

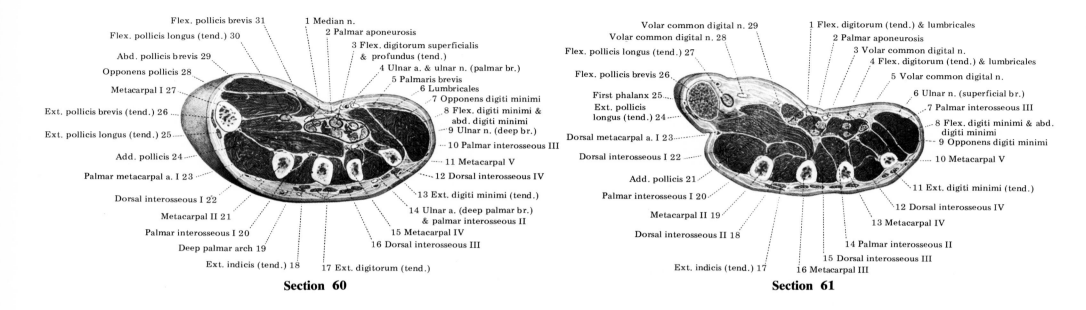

Flex. pollicis brevis 31
Flex. pollicis longus (tend.) 30
Abd. pollicis brevis 29
Opponens pollicis 28
Metacarpal I 27
Ext. pollicis brevis (tend.) 26
Ext. pollicis longus (tend.) 25
Add. pollicis 24
Palmar metacarpal a. I 23
Dorsal interosseous I 22
Metacarpal II 21
Palmar interosseous I 20
Deep palmar arch 19
Ext. indicis (tend.) 18

1 Median n.
2 Palmar aponeurosis
3 Flex. digitorum superficialis & profundus (tend.)
4 Ulnar a. & ulnar n. (palmar br.)
5 Palmaris brevis
6 Lumbricales
7 Opponens digiti minimi
8 Flex. digiti minimi & abd. digiti minimi
9 Ulnar n. (deep br.)
10 Palmar interosseous III
11 Metacarpal V
12 Dorsal interosseous IV
13 Ext. digiti minimi (tend.)
14 Ulnar a. (deep palmar br.) & palmar interosseous II
15 Metacarpal IV
16 Dorsal interosseous III
17 Ext. digitorum (tend.)

Section 60

Volar common digital n. 29
Volar common digital n. 28
Flex. pollicis longus (tend.) 27
Flex. pollicis brevis 26
First phalanx 25
Ext. pollicis longus (tend.) 24
Dorsal metacarpal a. I 23
Dorsal interosseous I 22
Add. pollicis 21
Palmar interosseous I 20
Metacarpal II 19
Dorsal interosseous II 18
Ext. indicis (tend.) 17

1 Flex. digitorum (tend.) & lumbricales
2 Palmar aponeurosis
3 Volar common digital n.
4 Flex. digitorum (tend.) & lumbricales
5 Volar common digital n.
6 Ulnar n. (superficial br.)
7 Palmar interosseous III
8 Flex. digiti minimi & abd. digiti minimi
9 Opponens digiti minimi
10 Metacarpal V
11 Ext. digiti minimi (tend.)
12 Dorsal interosseous IV
13 Metacarpal IV
14 Palmar interosseous II
15 Dorsal interosseous III
16 Metacarpal III

Section 61

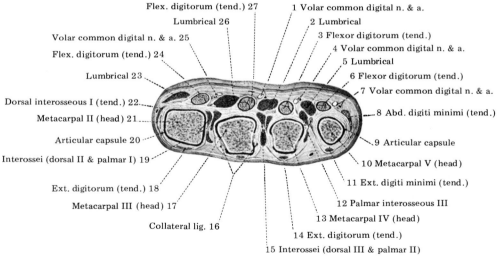

Flex. digitorum (tend.) 27
Lumbrical 26
Volar common digital n. & a. 25
Flex. digitorum (tend.) 24
Lumbrical 23
Dorsal interosseous I (tend.) 22
Metacarpal II (head) 21
Articular capsule 20
Interossei (dorsal II & palmar I) 19
Ext. digitorum (tend.) 18
Metacarpal III (head) 17
Collateral lig. 16

1 Volar common digital n. & a.
2 Lumbrical
3 Flexor digitorum (tend.)
4 Volar common digital n. & a.
5 Lumbrical
6 Flexor digitorum (tend.)
7 Volar common digital n. & a.
8 Abd. digiti minimi (tend.)
9 Articular capsule
10 Metacarpal V (head)
11 Ext. digiti minimi (tend.)
12 Palmar interosseous III
13 Metacarpal IV (head)
14 Ext. digitorum (tend.)
15 Interossei (dorsal III & palmar II)

Section 62

Volar common digital nn. 14
Flex. digitorum (tend.) 13
Phalanx I (digit II) 12
Extensor indicis (tend.) 11
Interosseous & lumbrical (tend.) 10
Ext. digitorum (tend.) 9
Interosseous & lumbrical (tend.) 8

1 Volar common digital aa.
2 Flex. digitorum (tend.)
3 Phalanx I (digit V)
4 Ext. digiti minimi (tend.)
5 Interosseous & lumbrical (tend.)
6 Phalanx I (digit IV)
7 Vaginal lig.

Section 63

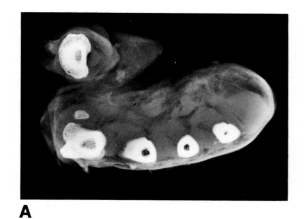

A

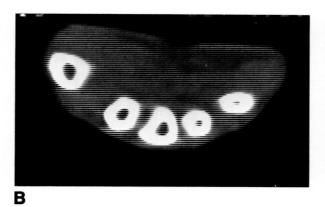

B

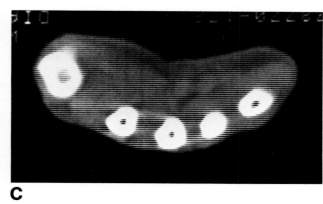

C

SECTIONS 60, 61, 62, 63

CT scans (**B**) and (**C**) and x-ray of specimen (**A**) are taken through the metacarpal bones revealing the flexor tendons, muscles of the hand and thumb, and the palmar fascia.

KEY FIGURES XII AND XIII These key figures represent a frontal view of the left leg. The bones and the principal arteries, veins, nerves, and muscles are shown. The levels of the following sections with reference to the various structures are indicated by the transverse lines 64–75.

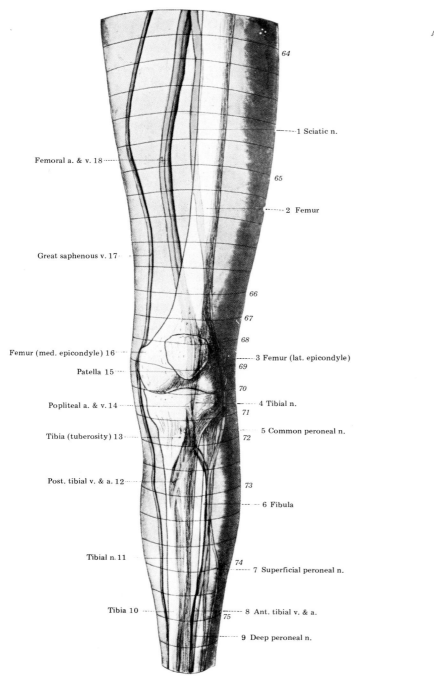

Femoral a. & v. 18

Great saphenous v. 17

Femur (med. epicondyle) 16

Patella 15

Popliteal a. & v. 14

Tibia (tuberosity) 13

Post. tibial v. & a. 12

Tibial n. 11

Tibia 10

1 Sciatic n.

64

65

2 Femur

66

67

68

3 Femur (lat. epicondyle)

69

70

4 Tibial n.

71

5 Common peroneal n.

72

73

6 Fibula

74

7 Superficial peroneal n.

8 Ant. tibial v. & a.

75

9 Deep peroneal n.

KEY FIGURE XII

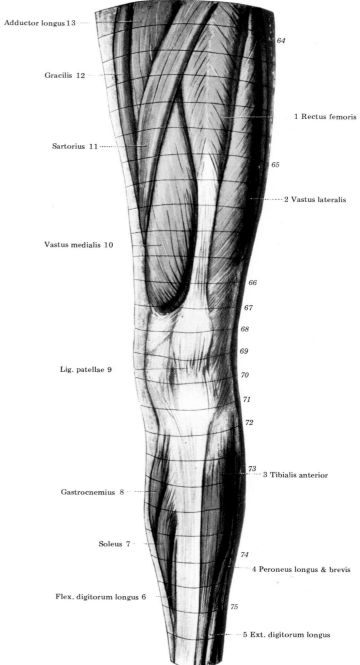

Adductor longus 13

Gracilis 12

Sartorius 11

Vastus medialis 10

Lig. patellae 9

Gastrocnemius 8

Soleus 7

Flex. digitorum longus 6

64

1 Rectus femoris

65

2 Vastus lateralis

66

67

68

69

70

71

72

73

3 Tibialis anterior

74

4 Peroneus longus & brevis

75

5 Ext. digitorum longus

KEY FIGURE XIII

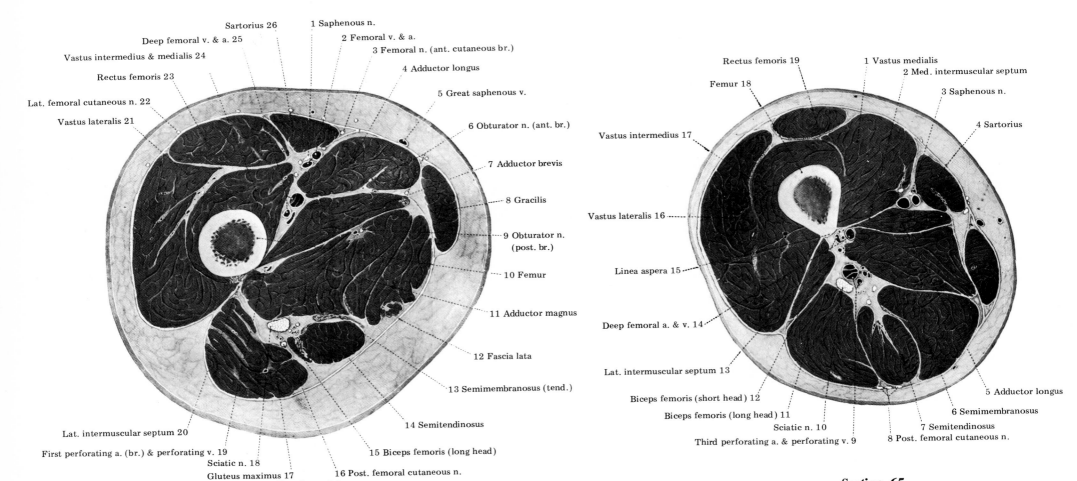

Sartorius 26
1 Saphenous n.
Deep femoral v. & a. 25
2 Femoral v. & a.
3 Femoral n. (ant. cutaneous br.)
Vastus intermedius & medialis 24
4 Adductor longus
Rectus femoris 23
5 Great saphenous v.
Lat. femoral cutaneous n. 22
6 Obturator n. (ant. br.)
Vastus lateralis 21
7 Adductor brevis
8 Gracilis
9 Obturator n. (post. br.)
10 Femur
11 Adductor magnus
12 Fascia lata
13 Semimembranosus (tend.)
Lat. intermuscular septum 20
14 Semitendinosus
First perforating a. (br.) & perforating v. 19
15 Biceps femoris (long head)
Sciatic n. 18
16 Post. femoral cutaneous n.
Gluteus maximus 17

Section 64

Rectus femoris 19
1 Vastus medialis
2 Med. intermuscular septum
Femur 18
3 Saphenous n.
4 Sartorius
Vastus intermedius 17
Vastus lateralis 16
Linea aspera 15
Deep femoral a. & v. 14
5 Adductor longus
Lat. intermuscular septum 13
6 Semimembranosus
Biceps femoris (short head) 12
7 Semitendinosus
Biceps femoris (long head) 11
8 Post. femoral cutaneous n.
Sciatic n. 10
Third perforating a. & perforating v. 9

Section 65

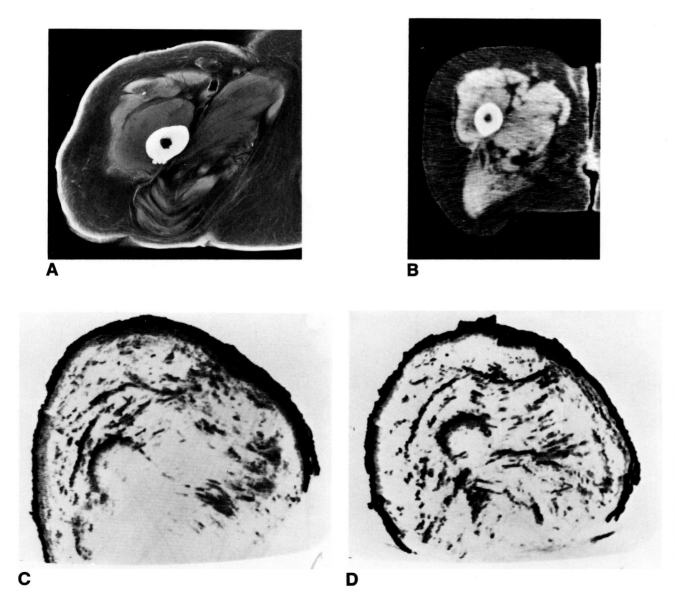

A

B

C

D

SECTIONS 64, 65

The femoral vessels are anteromedial to the femur, which is almost surrounded by the vastus muscle while the rectus femoris muscle can be seen anteriorly and the adductor muscles medially. These structures are all visible in the x-ray of the specimen (**A**), CT scan (**B**), and ultrasound (**C**) and (**D**). Sections (**A**) and (**B**) are of the proximal femur and show the gluteus maximus posteriorly. The last ultrasound (**D**) taken through the mid-femur shows the anterior rectus femoris sharply defined from the vastus muscle group, the lateral intermuscular septum inferolaterally. The biceps, semitendinous and semimembranous muscles are roughly outlined.

Quadriceps femoris (tend.) 19   1 Articularis genu

Vastus lateralis 18   2 Femur

Iliotibial tract 17   3 Vastus medialis

4 Popliteal surface

5 Adductor magnus (tend.)

6 Saphenous n.

7 Sartorius

8 Great saphenous v.

Biceps femoris 16   9 Gracilis

Variant v. 15

Tibial n. & common peroneal n. 14   10 Popliteal v. & a.

Small saphenous v. &
post. femoral cutaneous n. 13

Semimembranosus 12   11 Semitendinosus

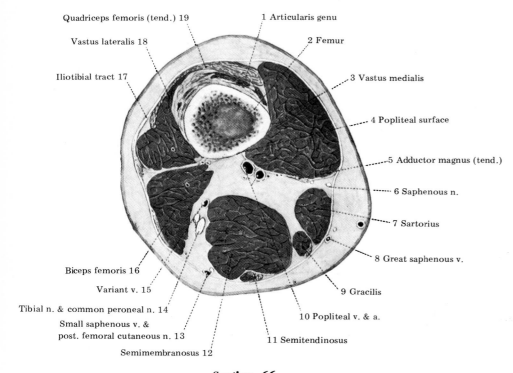

Section 66

Joint cavity 19   1 Quadriceps femoris (tend.)

Suprapatellar bursa 18   2 Popliteal v. & a.

3 Vastus medialis

Femur 17   4 Supreme genicular a.

Vastus lateralis 16   5 Adductor magnus (tend.)

Iliotibial tract 15

Biceps femoris 14   6 Saphenous n.

Popliteal surface 13   7 Great saphenous v.

Tibial n. & common peroneal n. 12   8 Gracilis (tend.) & sartorius

Small saphenous v. &
post. femoral cutaneous n. 11   9 Semitendinosus (tend.)

Semimembranosus 10

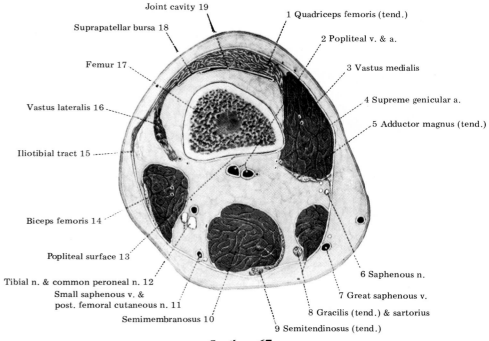

Section 67

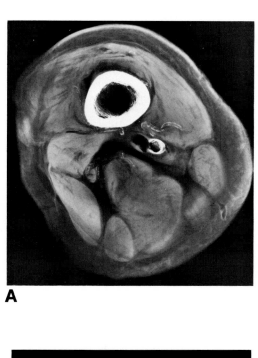

A

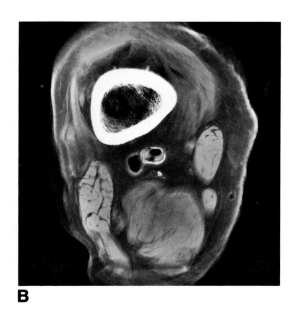

B

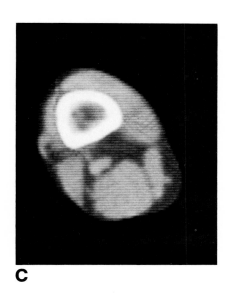

C

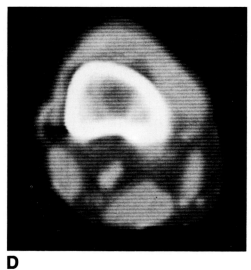

D

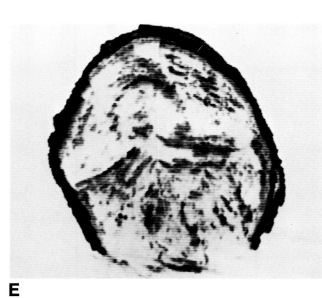

E

SECTIONS 66, 67

The popliteal vessels are readily identifiable posterior to the femur on the x-ray of the specimens (**A**) and (**B**) and CT scans (**C**) and (**D**). The medial and lateral vastus muscles largely surround the femur and are also evident on ultrasound (**C**). The lateral intermuscular septum and broader medial fascial plane are apparent. The semi-membranous muscle is encompassed by the biceps femoris and sartorius. The saphenous vein is also evident (**A**), (**B**), (**C**), and (**D**) in the subcutaneous tissue.

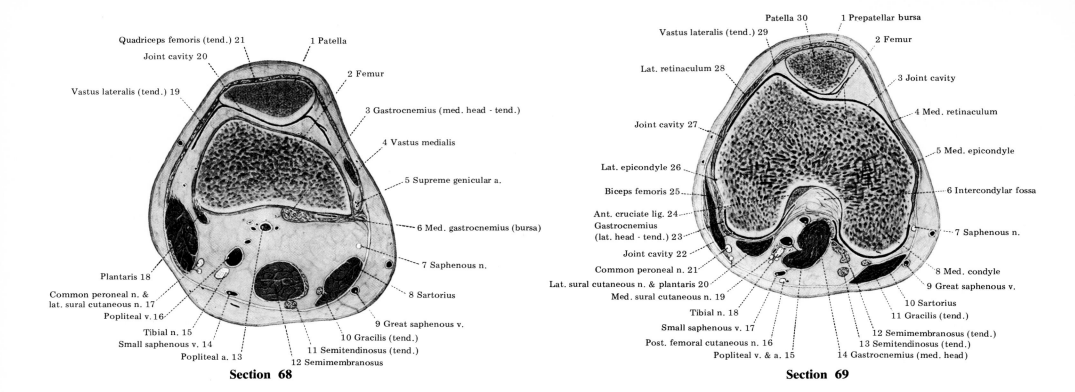

Quadriceps femoris (tend.) 21
Joint cavity 20
1 Patella
Vastus lateralis (tend.) 19
2 Femur
3 Gastrocnemius (med. head - tend.)
4 Vastus medialis
5 Supreme genicular a.
6 Med. gastrocnemius (bursa)
7 Saphenous n.
Plantaris 18
8 Sartorius
Common peroneal n. &
lat. sural cutaneous n. 17
Popliteal v. 16
9 Great saphenous v.
Tibial n. 15
10 Gracilis (tend.)
Small saphenous v. 14
11 Semitendinosus (tend.)
Popliteal a. 13
12 Semimembranosus

Section 68

Patella 30
1 Prepatellar bursa
Vastus lateralis (tend.) 29
2 Femur
Lat. retinaculum 28
3 Joint cavity
4 Med. retinaculum
Joint cavity 27
5 Med. epicondyle
Lat. epicondyle 26
6 Intercondylar fossa
Biceps femoris 25
7 Saphenous n.
Ant. cruciate lig. 24
Gastrocnemius
(lat. head - tend.) 23
Joint cavity 22
8 Med. condyle
Common peroneal n. 21
9 Great saphenous v.
Lat. sural cutaneous n. & plantaris 20
10 Sartorius
Med. sural cutaneous n. 19
11 Gracilis (tend.)
Tibial n. 18
12 Semimembranosus (tend.)
Small saphenous v. 17
13 Semitendinosus (tend.)
Post. femoral cutaneous n. 16
14 Gastrocnemius (med. head)
Popliteal v. & a. 15

Section 69

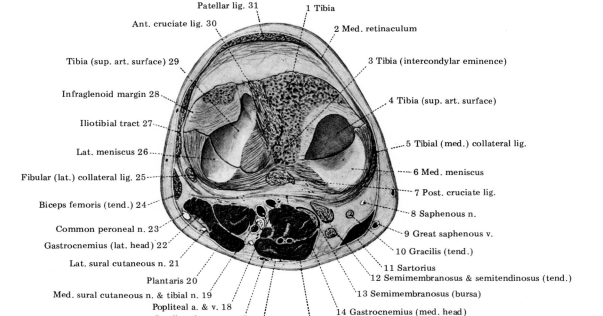

Patellar lig. 31
1 Tibia
Ant. cruciate lig. 30
2 Med. retinaculum
Tibia (sup. art. surface) 29
3 Tibia (intercondylar eminence)
Infraglenoid margin 28
4 Tibia (sup. art. surface)
Iliotibial tract 27
5 Tibial (med.) collateral lig.
Lat. meniscus 26
6 Med. meniscus
Fibular (lat.) collateral lig. 25
7 Post. cruciate lig.
Biceps femoris (tend.) 24
8 Saphenous n.
Common peroneal n. 23
9 Great saphenous v.
Gastrocnemius (lat. head) 22
10 Gracilis (tend.)
Lat. sural cutaneous n. 21
11 Sartorius
Plantaris 20
12 Semimembranosus & semitendinosus (tend.)
Med. sural cutaneous n. & tibial n. 19
13 Semimembranosus (bursa)
Popliteal a. & v. 18
14 Gastrocnemius (med. head)
Small saphenous v. 17
15 Articular capsule
Post. femoral cutaneous n. 16

Section 70

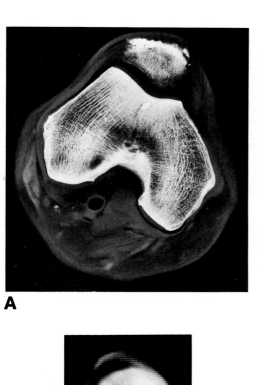

A

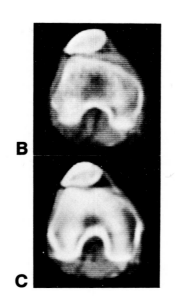

B

C

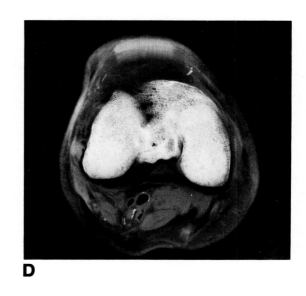

D

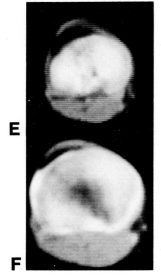

E

F

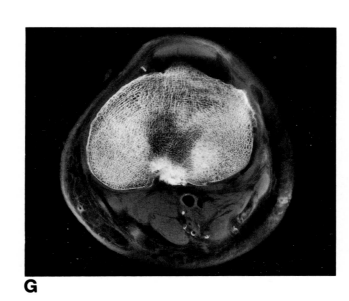

G

SECTIONS 68, 69, 70

Sections through the knee, as shown by x-rays of specimen (A), (D), (G), and CT scans (B), (C), (E), (F), reveal the patella, distal femur, and femoral condyles. The intercondylar eminence with the sites for the insertion of the cruciate ligaments is evident in (D). The tibial plateau and region of the medial and lateral menisci are seen in (E) and (F). Note the intercondylar fossa, the popliteal vessels, and the heads of the gastrocnemius muscle (G).

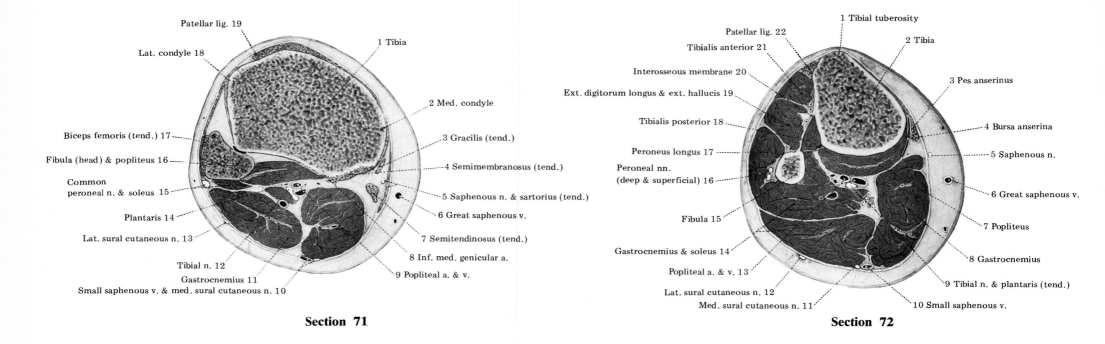

Patellar lig. 19

1 Tibia

Lat. condyle 18

2 Med. condyle

Biceps femoris (tend.) 17

3 Gracilis (tend.)

Fibula (head) & popliteus 16

4 Semimembranosus (tend.)

Common
peroneal n. & soleus 15

5 Saphenous n. & sartorius (tend.)

Plantaris 14

6 Great saphenous v.

Lat. sural cutaneous n. 13

7 Semitendinosus (tend.)

Tibial n. 12

8 Inf. med. genicular a.

Gastrocnemius 11

9 Popliteal a. & v.

Small saphenous v. & med. sural cutaneous n. 10

Section 71

1 Tibial tuberosity

Patellar lig. 22

2 Tibia

Tibialis anterior 21

Interosseous membrane 20

3 Pes anserinus

Ext. digitorum longus & ext. hallucis 19

4 Bursa anserina

Tibialis posterior 18

5 Saphenous n.

Peroneus longus 17

Peroneal nn.
(deep & superficial) 16

6 Great saphenous v.

Fibula 15

7 Popliteus

Gastrocnemius & soleus 14

8 Gastrocnemius

Popliteal a. & v. 13

9 Tibial n. & plantaris (tend.)

Lat. sural cutaneous n. 12

Med. sural cutaneous n. 11

10 Small saphenous v.

Section 72

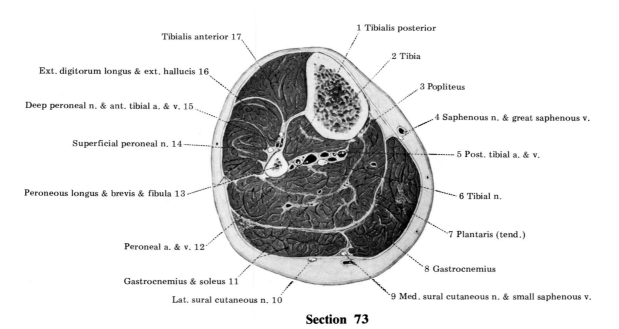

Tibialis anterior 17

1 Tibialis posterior

2 Tibia

Ext. digitorum longus & ext. hallucis 16

3 Popliteus

Deep peroneal n. & ant. tibial a. & v. 15

4 Saphenous n. & great saphenous v.

Superficial peroneal n. 14

5 Post. tibial a. & v.

Peroneous longus & brevis & fibula 13

6 Tibial n.

7 Plantaris (tend.)

Peroneal a. & v. 12

8 Gastrocnemius

Gastrocnemius & soleus 11

9 Med. sural cutaneous n. & small saphenous v.

Lat. sural cutaneous n. 10

Section 73

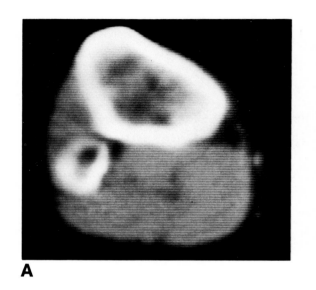

A

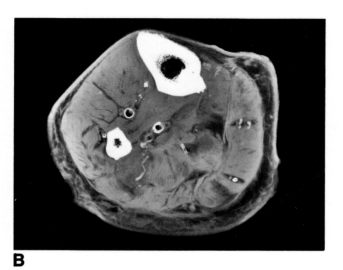

B

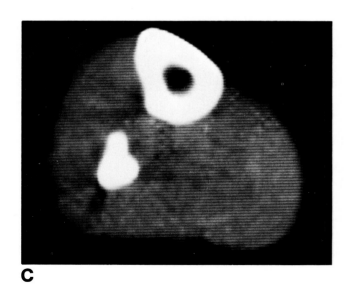

C

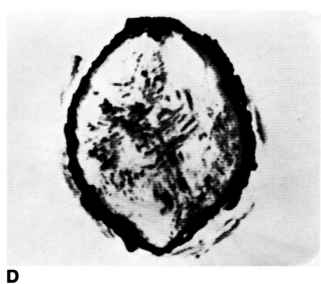

D

SECTIONS 71, 72, 73

The tibia, fibula, and interosseous membrane are visible on CT scans (**A**) and (**C**), X-ray of the specimen (**B**), and ultrasound (**D**). The muscle groups are more difficult to identify with less fat between the planes. The tibialis anterior lies lateral to the tibia; the gastrocnemius and soleus posterior to the bones. The saphenous veins are clearly seen in the subcutaneous tissue by CT scan (**A**).

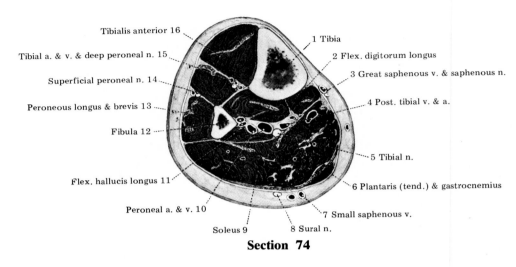

Tibialis anterior 16

Tibial a. & v. & deep peroneal n. 15

Superficial peroneal n. 14

Peroneous longus & brevis 13

Fibula 12

Flex. hallucis longus 11

Peroneal a. & v. 10

Soleus 9

8 Sural n.

7 Small saphenous v.

6 Plantaris (tend.) & gastrocnemius

5 Tibial n.

4 Post. tibial v. & a.

3 Great saphenous v. & saphenous n.

2 Flex. digitorum longus

1 Tibia

Section 74

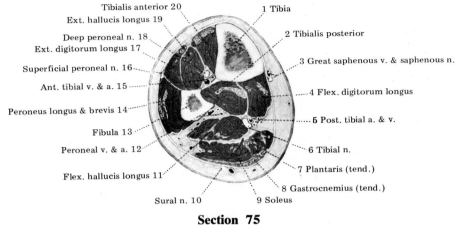

Tibialis anterior 20

Ext. hallucis longus 19

Deep peroneal n. 18

Ext. digitorum longus 17

Superficial peroneal n. 16

Ant. tibial v. & a. 15

Peroneus longus & brevis 14

Fibula 13

Peroneal v. & a. 12

Flex. hallucis longus 11

Sural n. 10

9 Soleus

8 Gastrocnemius (tend.)

7 Plantaris (tend.)

6 Tibial n.

5 Post. tibial a. & v.

4 Flex. digitorum longus

3 Great saphenous v. & saphenous n.

2 Tibialis posterior

1 Tibia

Section 75

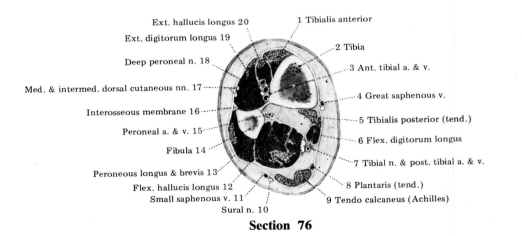

Ext. hallucis longus 20

Ext. digitorum longus 19

Deep peroneal n. 18

Med. & intermed. dorsal cutaneous nn. 17

Interosseous membrane 16

Peroneal a. & v. 15

Fibula 14

Peroneous longus & brevis 13

Flex. hallucis longus 12

Small saphenous v. 11

Sural n. 10

9 Tendo calcaneus (Achilles)

8 Plantaris (tend.)

7 Tibial n. & post. tibial a. & v.

6 Flex. digitorum longus

5 Tibialis posterior (tend.)

4 Great saphenous v.

3 Ant. tibial a. & v.

2 Tibia

1 Tibialis anterior

Section 76

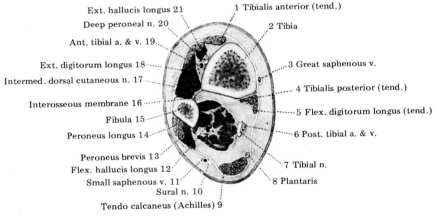

Ext. hallucis longus 21

Deep peroneal n. 20

Ant. tibial a. & v. 19

Ext. digitorum longus 18

Intermed. dorsal cutaneous n. 17

Interosseous membrane 16

Fibula 15

Peroneus longus 14

Peroneus brevis 13

Flex. hallucis longus 12

Small saphenous v. 11

Sural n. 10

Tendo calcaneus (Achilles) 9

8 Plantaris

7 Tibial n.

6 Post. tibial a. & v.

5 Flex. digitorum longus (tend.)

4 Tibialis posterior (tend.)

3 Great saphenous v.

2 Tibia

1 Tibialis anterior (tend.)

Section 77

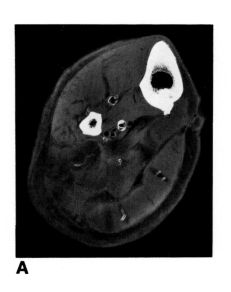

A

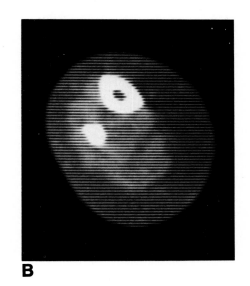

B

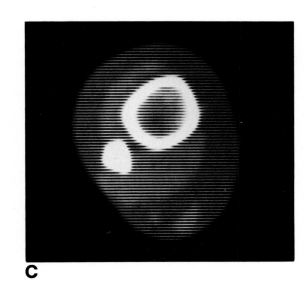

C

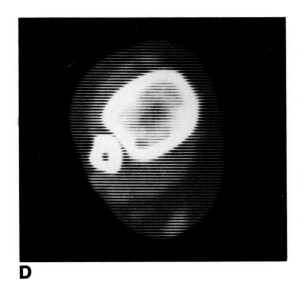

D

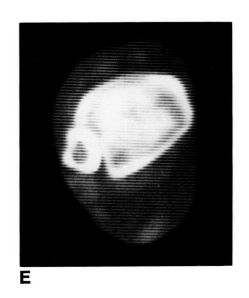

E

SECTIONS 74, 75, 76, 77

The bones, interosseous membrane and vessels are similar to the previous sections. Figure (**A**) is an x-ray of a specimen, and (**B-E**) are CT scans taken in sequence down toward the ankle. Note the Achilles tendon in (**D**) and (**E**).

KEY FIGURES XIV AND XV   These figures represent a side view of the foot and lower leg showing the position of the various bones as well as the principal ligaments and muscles. The levels of the following sections are indicated by the transverse lines 78–87.

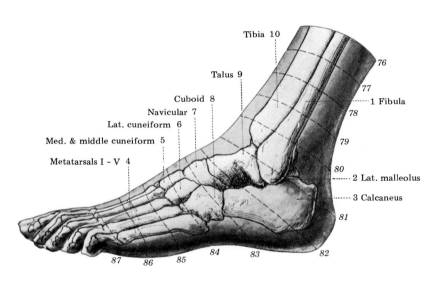

Tibia 10

Talus 9

Cuboid 8

Navicular 7

Lat. cuneiform 6

Med. & middle cuneiform 5

Metatarsals I - V 4

76

77

1 Fibula

78

79

80

2 Lat. malleolus

3 Calcaneus

81

82

87   86   85   84   83

KEY FIGURE XIV

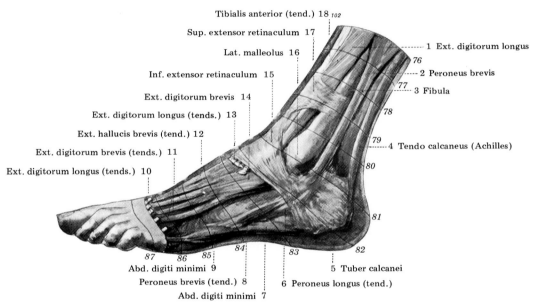

Tibialis anterior (tend.) 18 _102_

Sup. extensor retinaculum 17

Lat. malleolus 16

Inf. extensor retinaculum   15

Ext. digitorum brevis 14

Ext. digitorum longus (tends.) 13

Ext. hallucis brevis (tend.) 12

Ext. digitorum brevis (tends.) 11

Ext. digitorum longus (tends.) 10

1 Ext. digitorum longus

76

2 Peroneus brevis

77

3 Fibula

78

79

4 Tendo calcaneus (Achilles)

80

81

82

87   86   85   84   83

Abd. digiti minimi 9

Peroneus brevis (tend.) 8

Abd. digiti minimi 7

5 Tuber calcanei

6 Peroneus longus (tend.)

KEY FIGURE XV

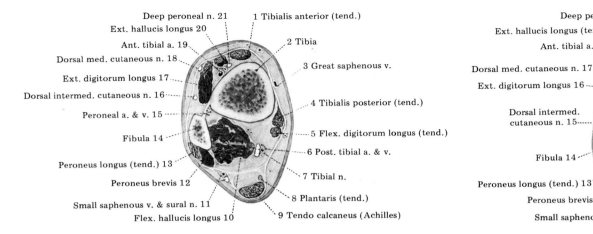

Deep peroneal n. 21
Ext. hallucis longus 20
Ant. tibial a. 19
Dorsal med. cutaneous n. 18
Ext. digitorum longus 17
Dorsal intermed. cutaneous n. 16
Peroneal a. & v. 15
Fibula 14
Peroneus longus (tend.) 13
Peroneus brevis 12
Small saphenous v. & sural n. 11
Flex. hallucis longus 10

1 Tibialis anterior (tend.)
2 Tibia
3 Great saphenous v.
4 Tibialis posterior (tend.)
5 Flex. digitorum longus (tend.)
6 Post. tibial a. & v.
7 Tibial n.
8 Plantaris (tend.)
9 Tendo calcaneus (Achilles)

Section 78

Deep peroneal n. 20
Ext. hallucis longus (tend.) 19
Ant. tibial a. 18
Dorsal med. cutaneous n. 17
Ext. digitorum longus 16
Dorsal intermed.
cutaneous n. 15
Fibula 14
Peroneus longus (tend.) 13
Peroneus brevis 12
Small saphenous v. 11

1 Tibialis anterior (tend.)
2 Great saphenous v.
3 Tibia
4 Tibialis posterior (tend.)
5 Flex. digitorum longus (tend.)
6 Flex. hallucis longus
7 Tibial n.
8 Post. tibial a. & v.
9 Plantaris (tend.)
10 Tendo calcaneus (Achilles)

Section 79

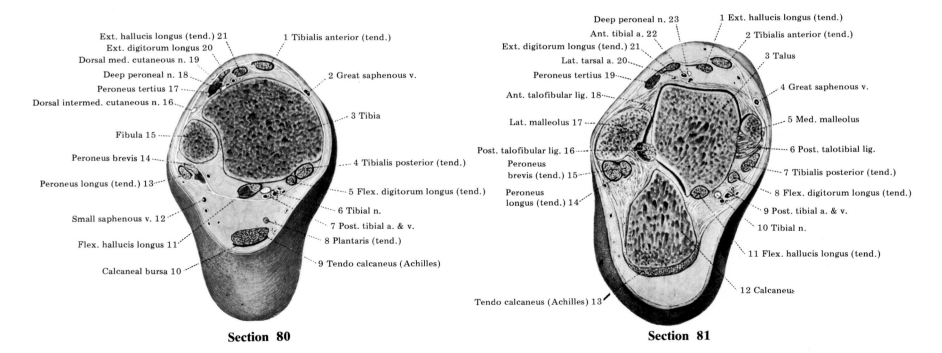

Ext. hallucis longus (tend.) 21
Ext. digitorum longus 20
Dorsal med. cutaneous n. 19
Deep peroneal n. 18
Peroneus tertius 17
Dorsal intermed. cutaneous n. 16
Fibula 15
Peroneus brevis 14
Peroneus longus (tend.) 13
Small saphenous v. 12
Flex. hallucis longus 11
Calcaneal bursa 10

1 Tibialis anterior (tend.)
2 Great saphenous v.
3 Tibia
4 Tibialis posterior (tend.)
5 Flex. digitorum longus (tend.)
6 Tibial n.
7 Post. tibial a. & v.
8 Plantaris (tend.)
9 Tendo calcaneus (Achilles)

Section 80

Deep peroneal n. 23
Ant. tibial a. 22
Ext. digitorum longus (tend.) 21
Lat. tarsal a. 20
Peroneus tertius 19
Ant. talofibular lig. 18
Lat. malleolus 17
Post. talofibular lig. 16
Peroneus
brevis (tend.) 15
Peroneus
longus (tend.) 14
Tendo calcaneus (Achilles) 13

1 Ext. hallucis longus (tend.)
2 Tibialis anterior (tend.)
3 Talus
4 Great saphenous v.
5 Med. malleolus
6 Post. talotibial lig.
7 Tibialis posterior (tend.)
8 Flex. digitorum longus (tend.)
9 Post. tibial a. & v.
10 Tibial n.
11 Flex. hallucis longus (tend.)
12 Calcaneus

Section 81

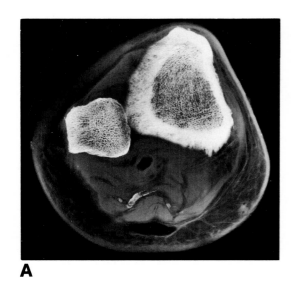

A

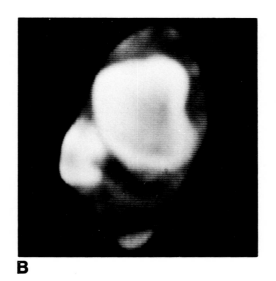

B

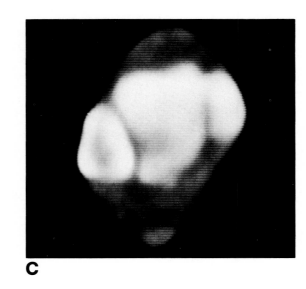

C

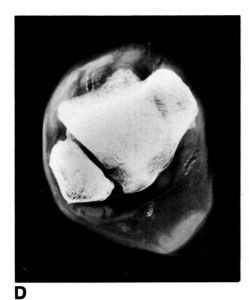

D

SECTIONS 78, 79, 80, 81

The bones about the ankle are visible on the x-ray of the specimen (**A**) and (**D**) and by CT scans (**B**) and (**C**). The medial and lateral malleoli (**C**) and (**D**), the talus (**C**), and achilles tendon are evident. The saphenous and other superficial veins can be seen in the subcutaneous tissue.

Sections 78, 79, 80, 81

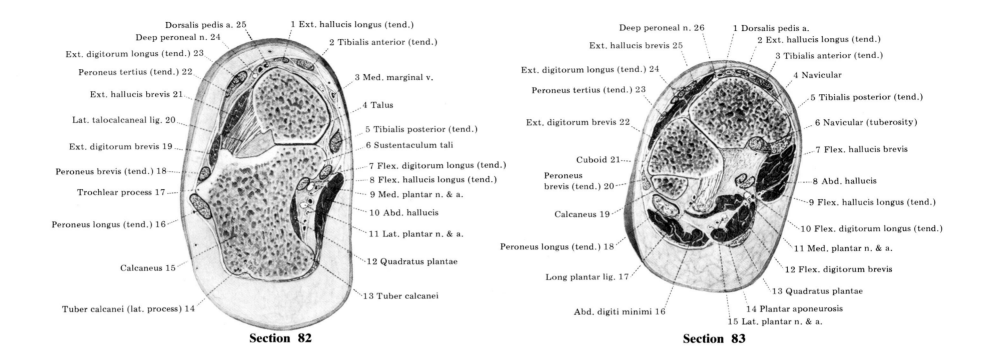

Section 82

Dorsalis pedis a. 25
Deep peroneal n. 24
Ext. digitorum longus (tend.) 23
Peroneus tertius (tend.) 22
Ext. hallucis brevis 21
Lat. talocalcaneal lig. 20
Ext. digitorum brevis 19
Peroneus brevis (tend.) 18
Trochlear process 17
Peroneus longus (tend.) 16
Calcaneus 15
Tuber calcanei (lat. process) 14

1 Ext. hallucis longus (tend.)
2 Tibialis anterior (tend.)
3 Med. marginal v.
4 Talus
5 Tibialis posterior (tend.)
6 Sustentaculum tali
7 Flex. digitorum longus (tend.)
8 Flex. hallucis longus (tend.)
9 Med. plantar n. & a.
10 Abd. hallucis
11 Lat. plantar n. & a.
12 Quadratus plantae
13 Tuber calcanei

Section 83

Deep peroneal n. 26
Ext. hallucis brevis 25
Ext. digitorum longus (tend.) 24
Peroneus tertius (tend.) 23
Ext. digitorum brevis 22
Cuboid 21
Peroneus brevis (tend.) 20
Calcaneus 19
Peroneus longus (tend.) 18
Long plantar lig. 17
Abd. digiti minimi 16

1 Dorsalis pedis a.
2 Ext. hallucis longus (tend.)
3 Tibialis anterior (tend.)
4 Navicular
5 Tibialis posterior (tend.)
6 Navicular (tuberosity)
7 Flex. hallucis brevis
8 Abd. hallucis
9 Flex. hallucis longus (tend.)
10 Flex. digitorum longus (tend.)
11 Med. plantar n. & a.
12 Flex. digitorum brevis
13 Quadratus plantae
14 Plantar aponeurosis
15 Lat. plantar n. & a.

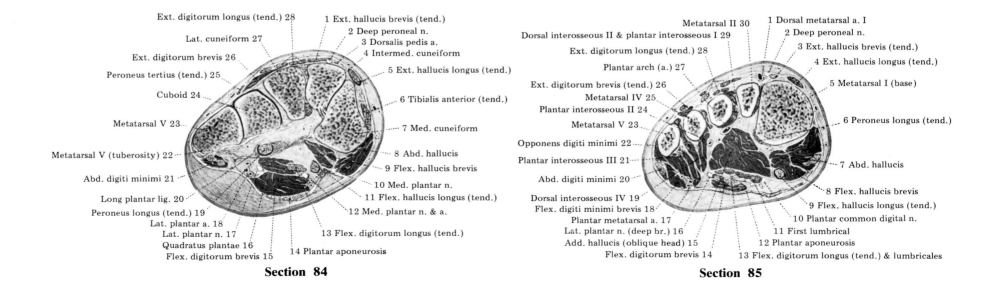

Section 84

Ext. digitorum longus (tend.) 28
Lat. cuneiform 27
Ext. digitorum brevis 26
Peroneus tertius (tend.) 25
Cuboid 24
Metatarsal V 23
Metatarsal V (tuberosity) 22
Abd. digiti minimi 21
Long plantar lig. 20
Peroneus longus (tend.) 19
Lat. plantar a. 18
Lat. plantar n. 17
Quadratus plantae 16
Flex. digitorum brevis 15

1 Ext. hallucis brevis (tend.)
2 Deep peroneal n.
3 Dorsalis pedis a.
4 Intermed. cuneiform
5 Ext. hallucis longus (tend.)
6 Tibialis anterior (tend.)
7 Med. cuneiform
8 Abd. hallucis
9 Flex. hallucis brevis
10 Med. plantar n.
11 Flex. hallucis longus (tend.)
12 Med. plantar n. & a.
13 Flex. digitorum longus (tend.)
14 Plantar aponeurosis

Section 85

Metatarsal II 30
Dorsal interosseous II & plantar interosseous I 29
Ext. digitorum longus (tend.) 28
Plantar arch (a.) 27
Ext. digitorum brevis (tend.) 26
Metatarsal IV 25
Plantar interosseous II 24
Metatarsal V 23
Opponens digiti minimi 22
Plantar interosseous III 21
Abd. digiti minimi 20
Dorsal interosseous IV 19
Flex. digiti minimi brevis 18
Plantar metatarsal a. 17
Lat. plantar n. (deep br.) 16
Add. hallucis (oblique head) 15
Flex. digitorum brevis 14

1 Dorsal metatarsal a. I
2 Deep peroneal n.
3 Ext. hallucis brevis (tend.)
4 Ext. hallucis longus (tend.)
5 Metatarsal I (base)
6 Peroneus longus (tend.)
7 Abd. hallucis
8 Flex. hallucis brevis
9 Flex. hallucis longus (tend.)
10 Plantar common digital n.
11 First lumbrical
12 Plantar aponeurosis
13 Flex. digitorum longus (tend.) & lumbricales

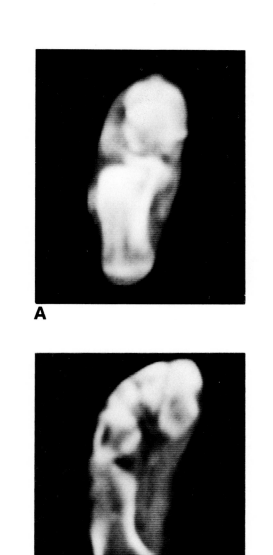

A

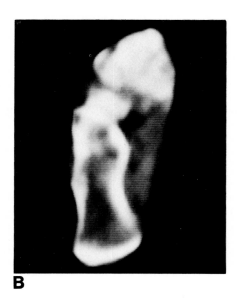

B

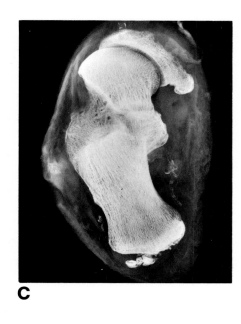

C

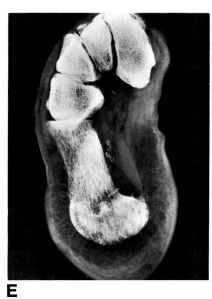

D

E

SECTIONS 82, 83, 84, 85

CT scans **(A)**, **(B)**, **(D)**, and x-rays of specimens **(C)** and **(E)** taken through the foot at an oblique angle show the os calcis; the talus **(A)** and **(C)**; the cuboid **(B)** and **(E)**; and the cuneiform bones **(D)** and **(E).** The normal soft tissue structures are difficult to identify.

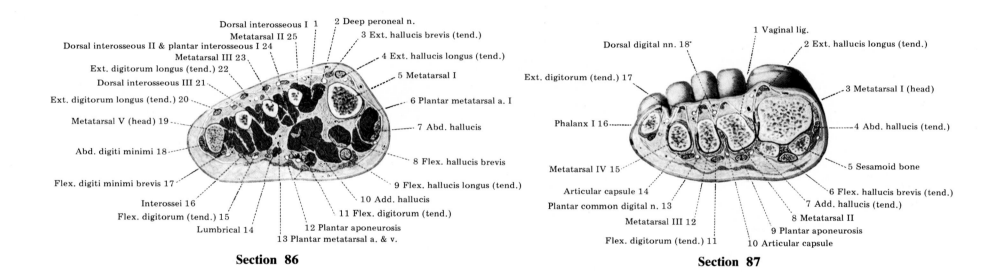

Dorsal interosseous I 1
Metatarsal II 25
Dorsal interosseous II & plantar interosseous I 24
Metatarsal III 23
Ext. digitorum longus (tend.) 22
Dorsal interosseous III 21
Ext. digitorum longus (tend.) 20
Metatarsal V (head) 19
Abd. digiti minimi 18
Flex. digiti minimi brevis 17
Interossei 16
Flex. digitorum (tend.) 15
Lumbrical 14

2 Deep peroneal n.
3 Ext. hallucis brevis (tend.)
4 Ext. hallucis longus (tend.)
5 Metatarsal I
6 Plantar metatarsal a. I
7 Abd. hallucis
8 Flex. hallucis brevis
9 Flex. hallucis longus (tend.)
10 Add. hallucis
11 Flex. digitorum (tend.)
12 Plantar aponeurosis
13 Plantar metatarsal a. & v.

Section 86

Dorsal digital nn. 18
Ext. digitorum (tend.) 17
Phalanx I 16
Metatarsal IV 15
Articular capsule 14
Plantar common digital n. 13
Metatarsal III 12
Flex. digitorum (tend.) 11

1 Vaginal lig.
2 Ext. hallucis longus (tend.)
3 Metatarsal I (head)
4 Abd. hallucis (tend.)
5 Sesamoid bone
6 Flex. hallucis brevis (tend.)
7 Add. hallucis (tend.)
8 Metatarsal II
9 Plantar aponeurosis
10 Articular capsule

Section 87

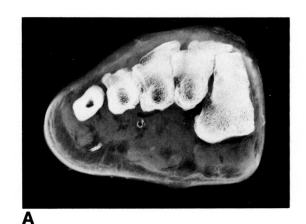

A

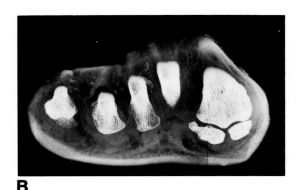

B

SECTIONS 86, 87

X-rays of sections through the foot show the base of the metatarsals (see Section 85), the plantar muscle and aponeurosis (A), and the relationship of the sesamoid bones (B) to the first metatarsal and the plantar arch.

SAGITTAL SECTIONS

In addition to the transverse sections, which can be produced by computed tomography and echography, sagittal sections can also be easily obtained with the use of the ultrasound beam. A series of representative sagittal sections through the abdomen are presented. The first five are done with the subject supine, and the last one with the subject prone. The cephalic structures are presented to the left.

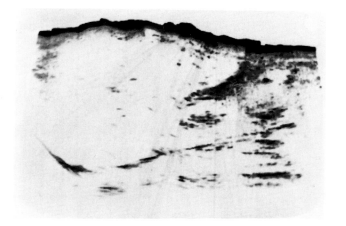

A sagittal section through the right side of the abdomen just lateral to the midclavicular line (**A**) demonstrates the liver, and shows the kidney close to the posterior surface of the right hepatic lobe. The direction of the plane is not perpendicular to the ultrasound beam, thus the separation of liver and kidney is not fully demonstrated. Below the liver, bowel loops present as uninterpretable aggregations of echoes.

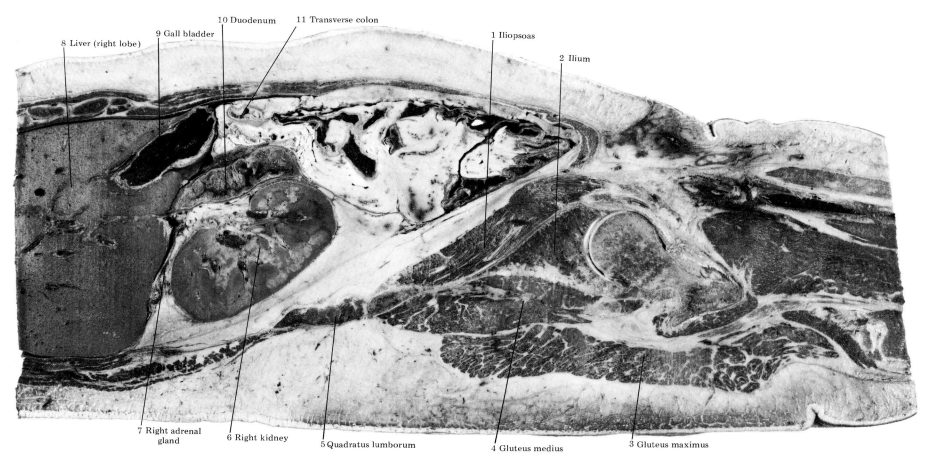

8 Liver (right lobe)

9 Gall bladder

10 Duodenum

11 Transverse colon

1 Iliopsoas

2 Ilium

7 Right adrenal gland

6 Right kidney

5 Quadratus lumborum

4 Gluteus medius

3 Gluteus maximus

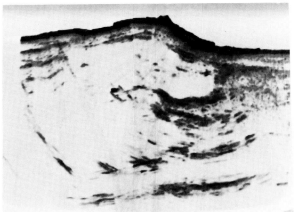

A section just medial to the midclavicular line (**B**) demonstrates the liver and diaphragm. The echo-free area anterior to the inferior surface of the liver is the gallbladder. The relatively sonolucent area in the same plane as the kidney on the previous section represents the psoas muscle extending to the caudal end of the picture.

Sagittal Sections

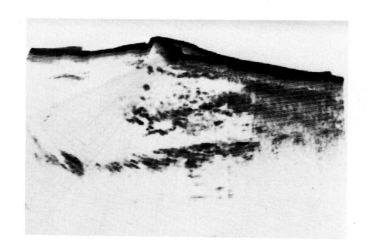

A section just to the right of the midline (**C**) shows the more pointed configuration of the left lobe of the liver anteriorly. The rounded structure just behind this is the portal vein. The inferior vena cava can be seen as a relatively echo-free area just anterior to the spine and behind the portal vein. The structure between the left lobe of the liver and the inferior vena cava represents a portion of the pancreas.

Sagittal Sections

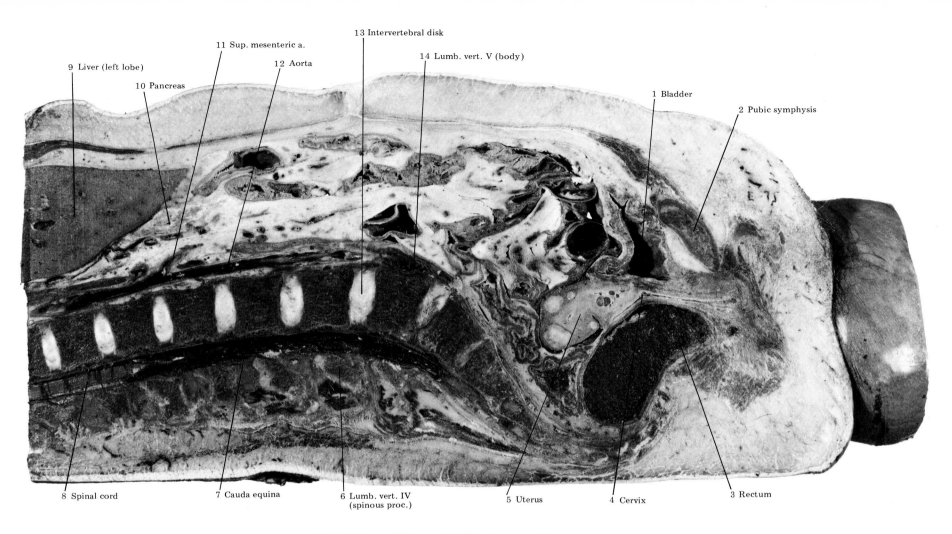

9 Liver (left lobe)

10 Pancreas

11 Sup. mesenteric a.

12 Aorta

13 Intervertebral disk

14 Lumb. vert. V (body)

1 Bladder

2 Pubic symphysis

8 Spinal cord

7 Cauda equina

6 Lumb. vert. IV (spinous proc.)

5 Uterus

4 Cervix

3 Rectum

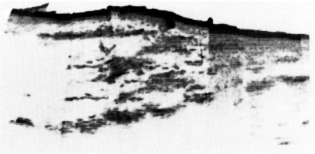

A section just to the left of the midline (**D**) shows the spine posteriorly and the aorta in front of the spine. The left lobe of the liver is seen anteriorly. The superior mesenteric artery can be faintly identified as a slightly curvilinear structure arising from the aorta and passing anteriorly and then inferiorly. Just in front of the superior mesenteric artery is a relatively echo-free area which represents the body of the pancreas.

Sagittal Sections

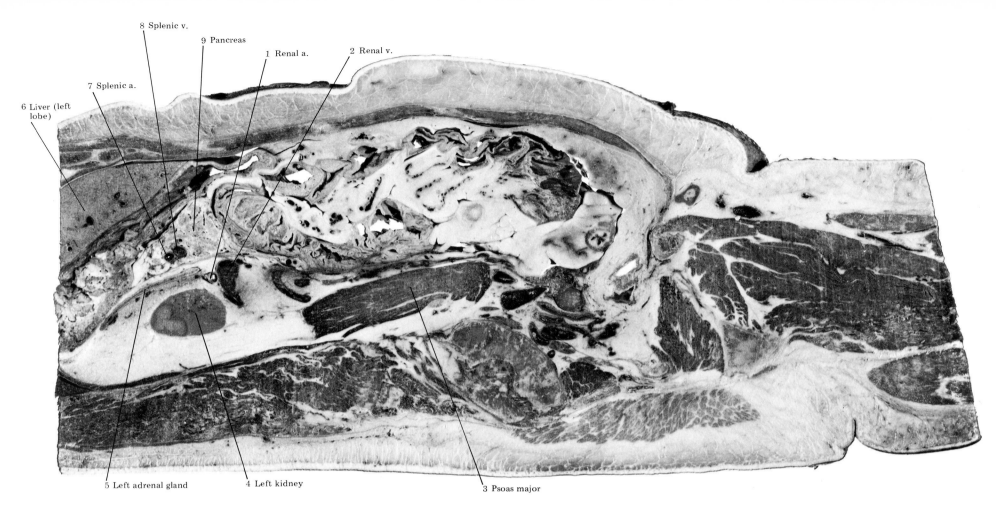

8 Splenic v.

9 Pancreas

1 Renal a.

2 Renal v.

7 Splenic a.

6 Liver (left lobe)

5 Left adrenal gland

4 Left kidney

3 Psoas major

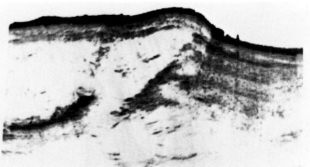

A sagittal section at the left midclavicular line (**E**) shows the small triangular shape of the left lobe of the liver. The diaphragm separates this from the cardiac contour. The posterior wall of the heart is particularly well shown. Below the level of the left lobe of the liver, the bowel activity obscures anatomic structures. The left side of the abdomen is difficult to study because of the large amount of gas-containing bowel normally located in this area.

Sagittal Sections

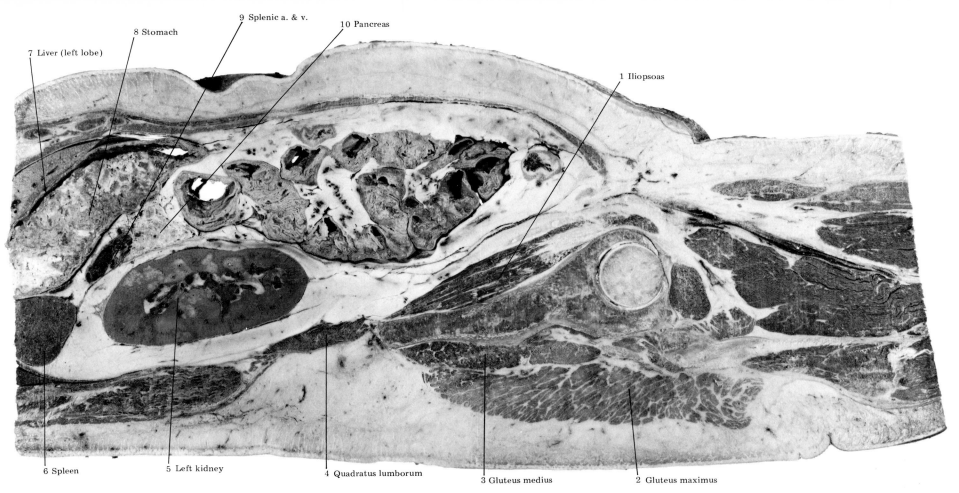

7 Liver (left lobe)

8 Stomach

9 Splenic a. & v.

10 Pancreas

1 Iliopsoas

6 Spleen

5 Left kidney

4 Quadratus lumborum

3 Gluteus medius

2 Gluteus maximus

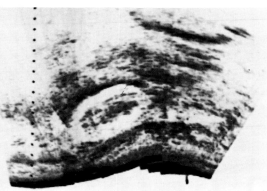

A prone section 7 cm to the left of the midline (**F**) demonstrates the left kidney as well as the psoas muscle below it. The spleen is seen as a sonolucent area near the top of the film. The presence of bowel gas obscures the other abdominal structures.

Sagittal Sections

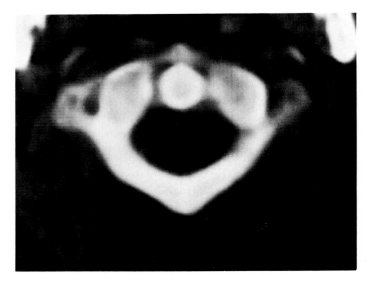

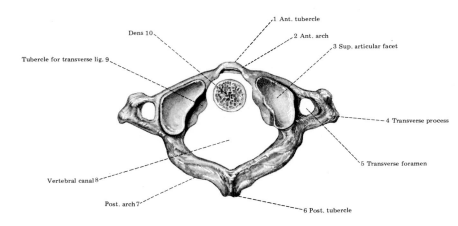

Dens 10

Tubercle for transverse lig. 9

Vertebral canal 8

Post. arch 7

1 Ant. tubercle

2 Ant. arch

3 Sup. articular facet

4 Transverse process

5 Transverse foramen

6 Post. tubercle

CERVICAL VERTEBRA C1 (A)

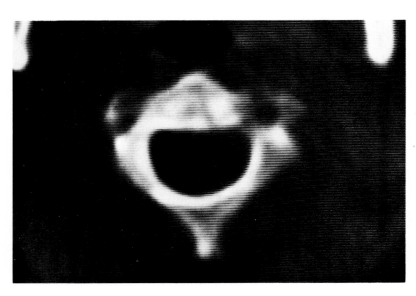

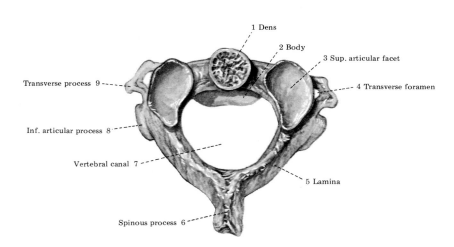

1 Dens

2 Body

3 Sup. articular facet

4 Transverse foramen

Transverse process 9

Inf. articular process 8

Vertebral canal 7

5 Lamina

Spinous process 6

CERVICAL VERTEBRA C2 (B)

Cervical Spine

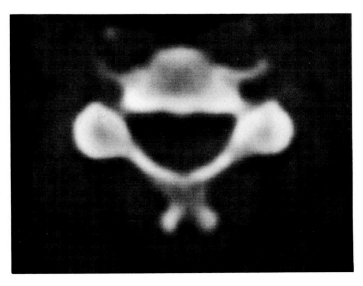

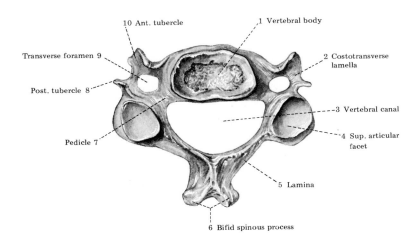

10 Ant. tubercle

1 Vertebral body

Transverse foramen 9

2 Costotransverse lamella

Post. tubercle 8

3 Vertebral canal

Pedicle 7

4 Sup. articular facet

5 Lamina

6 Bifid spinous process

CERVICAL VERTEBRA C4 (C)

CERVICAL SPINE

Section diagrams and corresponding scans of cervical vertebrae CI, C2, and C4 are shown. These scans and diagrams should be correlated with the sections (**A**), (**B**), (**C**), as illustrated in the lateral line drawing (left). Note that the entire dens is not seen in C1 and C2 since sections (**A**) and (**B**) are only 13 mm thick.

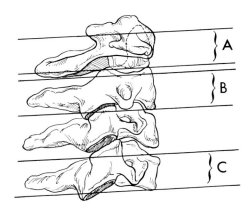

A

B

C

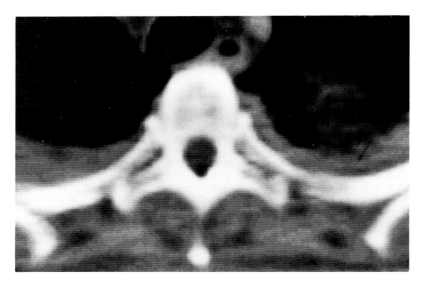

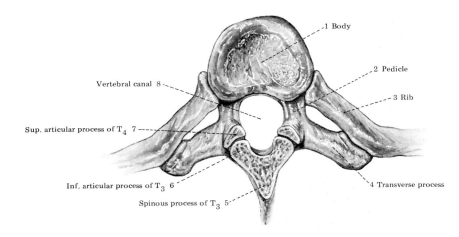

1 Body

2 Pedicle

3 Rib

4 Transverse process

Vertebral canal 8

Sup. articular process of T$_4$ 7

Inf. articular process of T$_3$ 6

Spinous process of T$_3$ 5

DORSAL VERTEBRA T4 (A)

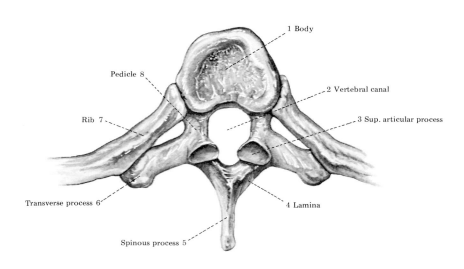

1 Body

Pedicle 8

2 Vertebral canal

Rib 7

3 Sup. articular process

Transverse process 6

4 Lamina

Spinous process 5

Dorsal Spine

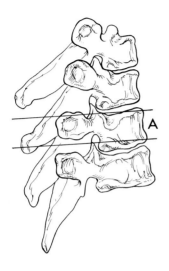

A

DORSAL SPINE

The scan is of dorsal vertebra T4. Two diagrams are shown. The section diagram on the top left correlates with a 13 mm thick section and therefore includes part of the body of T4 and spinous process of T3 (see lateral line drawing above, Section **A**). The anatomic diagram on the bottom left is a superior view of a disarticulated T4 with the adjacent ribs.

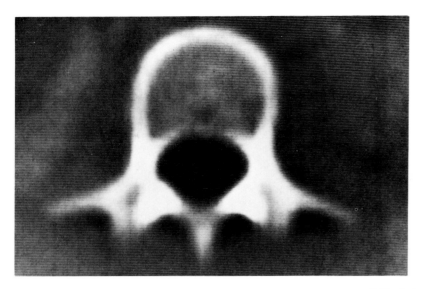

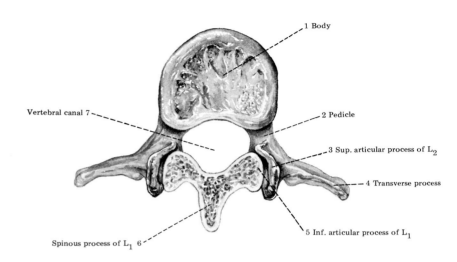

1 Body

Vertebral canal 7

2 Pedicle

3 Sup. articular process of L$_2$

4 Transverse process

5 Inf. articular process of L$_1$

Spinous process of L$_1$ 6

LUMBAR VERTEBRA L2 (A)

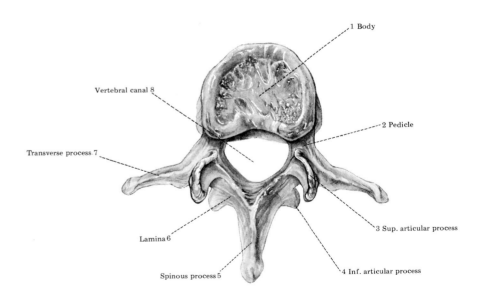

1 Body

Vertebral canal 8

2 Pedicle

Transverse process 7

3 Sup. articular process

Lamina 6

4 Inf. articular process

Spinous process 5

Upper Lumbar Spine

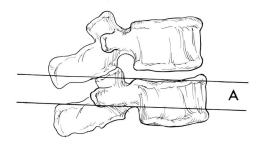

UPPER LUMBAR SPINE

The scan is of lumbar vertebra L2. Two diagrams are shown. The section diagram on the top left correlates with a 13 mm thick section and therefore includes most of the body of L2 together with part of the spinous process and inferior articular processes of L1 (see lateral line drawing above, Section **A**). The anatomic diagram on the lower left is a superior view of a disarticulated L2.

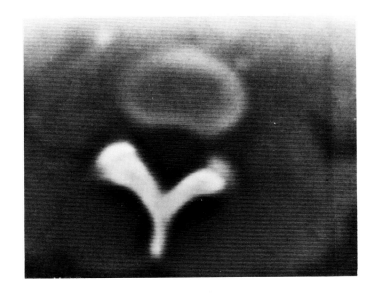

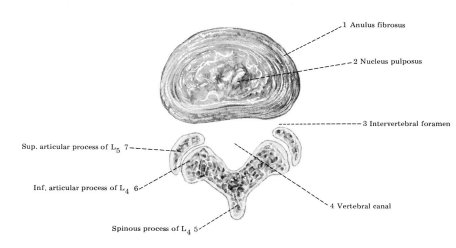

1 Anulus fibrosus

2 Nucleus pulposus

3 Intervertebral foramen

Sup. articular process of L₅ 7

Inf. articular process of L₄ 6

4 Vertebral canal

Spinous process of L₄ 5

L4-L5 DISC (A)

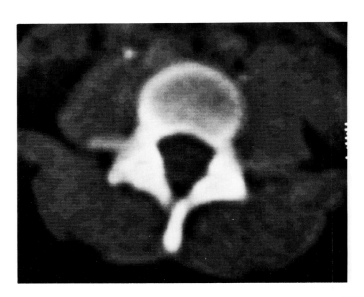

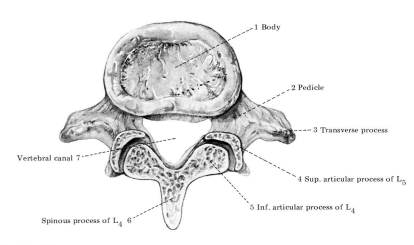

1 Body

2 Pedicle

3 Transverse process

Vertebral canal 7

4 Sup. articular process of L₅

5 Inf. articular process of L₄

Spinous process of L₄ 6

LUMBAR VERTEBRA L5 (B)

Lower Lumbar Spine

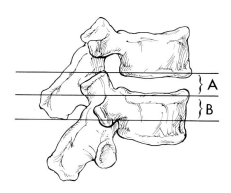

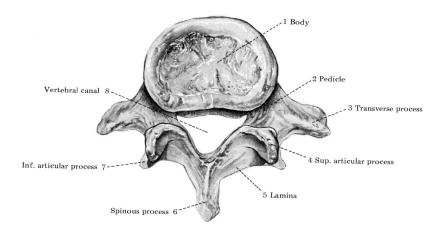

1 Body

2 Pedicle

3 Transverse process

4 Sup. articular process

5 Lamina

Spinous process 6

Inf. articular process 7

Vertebral canal 8

LOWER LUMBAR SPINE

The scan and illustration (top left) are of the intervertebral disc L4-L5, and this level includes part of the spinous process and inferior articular processes of L4 and parts of the superior articular processes of L5 (see lateral line drawing above left, Section **A**). The scan and illustration (bottom left) is of the upper part of the body of L5 and includes part of the spinous process and inferior articular processes of L4 (see lateral line drawing above left, Section **B**). The anatomic diagram (above right) is a superior view of a disarticulated L5. Note that using a 13 mm collimator, a scan through an intervertebral disc will include part of the adjacent vertebral end plates.

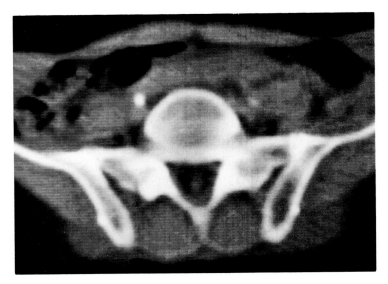

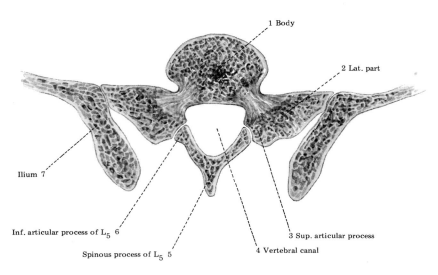

1 Body

2 Lat. part

Ilium 7

Inf. articular process of L$_5$ 6

Spinous process of L$_5$ 5

4 Vertebral canal

3 Sup. articular process

SACRAL VERTEBRA S1 (A)

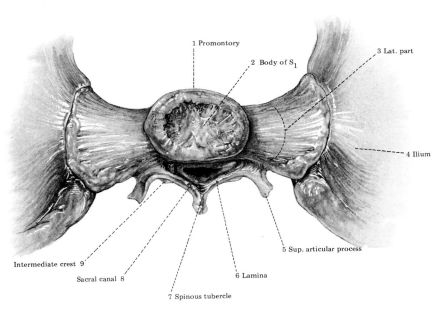

1 Promontory

2 Body of S$_1$

3 Lat. part

4 Ilium

5 Sup. articular process

6 Lamina

7 Spinous tubercle

Sacral canal 8

Intermediate crest 9

Upper Sacrum

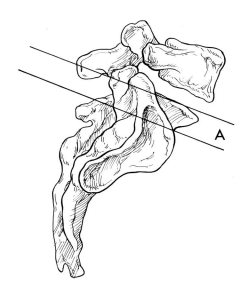

A

UPPER SACRUM

The scan and illustration (top left) are of the upper part of S1 and adjacent sacroiliac joint. The section diagram includes the body and lateral part of S1, part of the spinous process and inferior articular processes of L5 and the medial aspects of the iliac bones (see lateral line drawing above, Section **A**). The anatomic drawing (bottom left) is a superior view of a disarticulated sacrum and adjacent iliac bones.

Index

Each entry is followed by two numbers that are separated by a dash. The first number refers to the Section where that entry can be found, the second number refers to the item in that Section. For example, in the first entry the acetabulum can be found in Section 39, item 55 and Section 45, item 43. Roman numerals refer to Key Figures and the letter "S" refers to the Sagittal sections.